W9-BKF-949

Also by Vijay Vad

BACK RX

GOLF RX (with Dave Allen)

# ARTHRITIS Rx

## A CUTTING-EDGE PROGRAM
## FOR A PAIN-FREE LIFE

Vijay Vad, M.D.

GOTHAM
BOOKS

GOTHAM BOOKS
Published by Penguin Group (USA) Inc.
375 Hudson Street, New York, New York 10014, U.S.A.

Penguin Group (Canada), 90 Eglinton Avenue East, Suite 700, Toronto, Ontario M4P 2Y3, Canada (a division of Pearson Penguin Canada Inc.); Penguin Books Ltd, 80 Strand, London WC2R 0RL, England; Penguin Ireland, 25 St Stephen's Green, Dublin 2, Ireland (a division of Penguin Books Ltd); Penguin Group (Australia), 250 Camberwell Road, Camberwell, Victoria 3124, Australia (a division of Pearson Australia Group Pty Ltd); Penguin Books India Pvt Ltd, 11 Community Centre, Panchsheel Park, New Delhi - 110 017, India; Penguin Group (NZ), cnr Airborne and Rosedale Roads, Albany, Auckland 1310, New Zealand (a division of Pearson New Zealand Ltd); Penguin Books (South Africa) (Pty) Ltd, 24 Sturdee Avenue, Rosebank, Johannesburg 2196, South Africa

Penguin Books Ltd, Registered Offices: 80 Strand, London WC2R 0RL, England

Published by Gotham Books, a division of Penguin Group (USA) Inc.

Previously published as a Gotham Book hardcover edition, April 2006

First trade paperback printing, March 2007

10   9   8   7   6   5   4   3   2

Copyright © 2006 by Vijay Vad
Photographs © 2006 by McLain Bennett
All rights reserved

Gotham Books and the skyscraper logo are trademarks of Penguin Group (USA) Inc.

The Library of Congress has cataloged the hardcover edition as follows:
Vad, Vijay.
    Arthritis Rx : a cutting-edge program for a pain-free life / Vijay Vad.
       p.   cm.
    ISBN 1-592-40164-3 (hardcover)    ISBN 978-1-592-40274-8 (paperback)
    1. Arthritis—Treatment.   2. Arthritis—Alternative treatment.   I. Title.
    RC933.V33   2006
    616.7'2206—dc22      2005023915

Printed in the United States of America
Set in Electra

Without limiting the rights under copyright reserved above, no part of this publication may be reproduced, stored in, or introduced into a retrieval system, or transmitted, in any form, or by any means (electronic, mechanical, photocopying, recording, or otherwise), without the prior written permission of both the copyright owner and the above publisher of this book.

The scanning, uploading, and distribution of this book via the Internet or via any other means without the permission of the publisher is illegal and punishable by law. Please purchase only authorized electronic editions, and do not participate in or encourage electronic piracy of copyrighted materials. Your support of the author's rights is appreciated.

While the author has made every effort to provide accurate telephone numbers and Internet addresses at the time of publication, neither the publisher nor the author assumes any responsibility for errors, or for changes that occur after publication. Further, the publisher does not have any control over and does not assume any responsibility for author or third-party Web sites or their content.

I dedicate this book to my grandfather Gangadhar M. Vad, whose spirit lives on through the Vad Foundation, which is dedicated to world peace and prosperity by educating disadvantaged children and enhancing the quality of life through medical research.

# CONTENTS

# ACKNOWLEDGMENTS

I would like to thank Chris Godek, whose wisdom and insight guided me through this project; Peter Occhiogrosso, who did a spectacular job in revising the manuscript; Sharon Johnson for her hard work in helping compile the first draft of the manuscript; my agent, Stuart Krichevsky, for his unfailing support and diligence; McLain Bennett, for her work on the photographs; William Cahill, who took the cover photo, and my talented wife, Dilshaad, who put together the Arthritis Rx recipes. Thanks also to Wendy Huntington and Kelly Griffin for their assistance with research.

Gotham Books is fortunate to have an amazing group of publishers. Thanks especially to William Shinker, who has strongly believed in and supported our vision; Lauren Marino for doing a fantastic job as editor; Sabrina Bowers and Ray Lundgren for great work with the interior and cover; and Hilary Terrell for coordinating the many elements involved in the process.

# FOREWORD

Joint pain caused by arthritis is among the most common reasons patients consult their physicians. It is also a leading reason that people decrease physical activity and experience less joy in life. But there is a great deal one can do to prevent arthritis from interfering with an active and productive life.

This book focuses on arthritis—in its most common form—but the information is relevant to those who suffer from any of the other one hundred types of arthritis. Within these pages, you will find practical advice that you can use to manage your condition whether you have been recently diagnosed or have battled arthritis for decades.

Explaining arthritis is not an easy task; there is much we need to learn about its cause and how to halt or delay its progress. This book explains the disease clearly and succinctly, capitalizing on Dr. Vijay Vad's extensive clinical experience and research. He provides the latest information about management fundamentals and what role a healthy lifestyle plays in maintaining joint function.

What is uniquely valuable about Dr. Vad's Arthritis Rx Plan—which combines an in-depth anti-inflammatory diet, nutritional supplements, and a series of exercises based on yoga and Pilates—is his step-by-step directions. Although his knowledge and experience are both comprehensive and exhaustive, his approach is minimalist. He consistently advocates the least invasive, least complicated, and least costly treatment at each step of the way. He allows readers to take charge of their own healing process as much as possible. Experts in nutrition, physical therapy, and other areas assisted in the discussion of treatment options. But in the end, it is up to the individual, in consultation with his or her physician, to do what is necessary to break the grip arthritis has on his or her life. I believe that if you use the strategies in this book, you will be able to continue to enjoy life and all the activities you do.

—Thomas P. Sculco, Board Member, Arthritis Foundation;
and Surgeon-in-Chief, Hospital for Special Surgery

# INTRODUCTION

As a young child I observed firsthand the debilitating effects that arthritis had on my grandfather Gangadhar Vad, who battled the disease for the last two decades of his life. Grandpa Vad graduated from the Royal Institute of Science of Bombay University and loved playing field hockey and tennis, but in his thirties a hockey injury to his knee was critical in instigating the early onset of arthritis. Later in life, that knee lost its shock-absorbing capabilities, resulting in chronic pain and stiffness. I saw how arthritis threatened to rob my grandfather of his vitality and vigor. At the same time, I saw how determined he was not to give in; he applied the discipline he had developed as a scholar to doing proper exercises and eating a healthy diet to maintain his mobility. As a child I was fascinated by his daily yoga routine and the elegant stretches he did to maintain the flexibility in his knee. He also ate fresh ginger daily, which the ancient Indian system of medicine known as Ayurveda counted as an effective treatment for arthritis. Only now is it being studied in Western medicine, with very encouraging results for reducing arthritis pain. My grandfather took thirty-minute walks daily to keep his body weight in check. His common-sense approach to managing knee arthritis kept him mobile enough to travel around the world at the ripe old age of eighty-five.

The oldest known chronic disease, arthritis harms the joints that connect our bones and enable us to move with ease. Arthritis is the nation's leading cause of disability among Americans over age fifteen and is second only to heart disease as a cause of workplace disability. In 1998 the number of people suffering from some form of arthritis was 43 million, or 1 in 6 Americans of all ages. The number of Americans currently battling all forms of arthritis or chronic joint symptoms tops 66 million, or 1 in 3 adults. Of that number, 25 million have osteoarthritis, which is the most common form of arthritis. Osteoarthritis is a degenerative disease in which the cartilage that covers the ends of bones in the joint deteriorates, causing pain and loss of movement as bones rub against each other. Rheumatoid arthritis, an autoimmune disease in which the joint lining becomes inflamed as part of the body's immune system activity, afflicts more than 3 million Americans, mostly women. In all, there are about one hundred forms of arthritis, including gout, lupus, sclerodoma, and psoriatic arthritis. But because so many more people suffer with osteoarthritis (numbers that will soar by 2030, as 76 million baby boomers born between 1946 and 1964 are now entering middle age, the time when the condition becomes more prevalent), this book focuses primarily on osteoarthritis. My Arthritis Rx Plan has been developed specifically for people afflicted with osteoarthritis. For convenience, I will use the term "arthritis" throughout to refer to osteoarthritis.

The pain of arthritis takes a heavy toll. Government health surveys have found that hip and knee pain is on the rise in older Americans. About 20 percent of men and 25 percent of women experience persistent knee pain every day. Another 12 percent of men and 16 percent of women battle hip pain. Younger people are affected, too. Arthritis of the hip, knee, and other joints causes many to give up playing sports and other activities.

But the good news is that today arthritis can be effectively managed. You can be spared the pain and disability that have sidelined millions in the past. This book emphasizes a take-charge approach to managing pain, stiffness, and other symptoms successfully through a simple, three-pronged approach. The Arthritis Rx Plan presents a complete regimen created around exercise, diet, and supplements. In the course of laying out my program, I also give you detailed information about proper breathing, nutrition, and weight control, and describe the latest advances in medications, physical therapy, and other treatment options. Using these strategies together with the guidance of your personal physician will enable you to limit the impact of arthritis so that you can enjoy an active, independent life.

As a physician specializing in sports medicine at the Hospital for Special Surgery and a professor at Weill Medical College of Cornell University in Manhattan, I have seen a revolution in the treatment of arthritis. When I entered medical school in the 1990s, there were few treatment options to alleviate symptoms. Most patients simply did physical therapy and took oral medications. If these measures were unsuccessful, the physician recommended total joint replacement, a surgical procedure to replace a worn-out knee, hip, or other damaged joint with a mechanical joint.

Along with other researchers, I began looking for middle ground—less invasive treatments and better diagnostic techniques—so that we could tailor treatments to the patient's specific needs. Now our research is reaping rewards: Many patients are able to control their pain with less invasive procedures. I was privileged to be trained at the Hospital for Special Surgery, which has been a pioneer in arthritis care for over one hundred fifty years. The first hip replacement in the United States was performed at our hospital, which also carried out hip replacement procedures for Pope John Paul II. The staff members here also recently pioneered the minimally invasive knee replacement. My educators and mentors at the hospital instilled the researcher and pioneer instincts in me. Because of this training and the immense research facilities and support network at the hospital, during the first three years of my practice I was able to do in-depth clinical studies on the role of an artificial-joint lubricant called hylan and its role in treating arthritis. My research in knee arthritis showed that the success rate of injecting hylan increases from 50 percent at one year to 80 percent at one year if a joint lavage is performed prior to instillation of this artificial lubricant. A joint lavage is a simple, non-surgical procedure that takes fifteen minutes and results in a clean joint devoid of arthritic debris with immediately increased flexibility and some degree of pain relief.

The knee arthritis studies were followed by a study on the arthritic hip that showed similar results. Both studies were published in 2003 in the prestigious peer-review journal *Archives of Physical Medicine and Rehabilitation*. I have successfully treated over five thousand arthritic hips and knees since then in this protocol that combines the joint lavage with injections of hylan. These technologies have delayed the need for joint replacement in the vast majority of treated patients, while reducing pain significantly and increasing mobility with a minimally invasive, non-surgical approach.

Once I had finished this research, I had the unique opportunity to travel with my wife to present my arthritis research to leading institutions around the world as a visiting professor through an educational grant. More important, I had the privilege of meeting renowned physicians and opinion leaders from Tokyo, Shanghai, Los Angeles, Boston, London, Switzerland, Germany, Italy, France, India, and Singapore. As I learned different ways of approaching arthritis from them, I also began to understand that our sedentary lifestyle, with minimal exercise and a highly processed diet full of refined sugar and fat, has contributed significantly to the vast projected increase in arthritis.

After spending so much time with medical leaders in arthritis from around the world, I came away convinced that we needed to have a more comprehensive solution for combating this major disease that robs the world's population of quality of life. I saw that as physicians, not only did we need to develop more minimally invasive technologies and better joint replacement, but we also had to come up with a more comprehensive basic solution to treat all of the population afflicted with arthritis at any stage of the disease. This basic solution had to address proper diet and exercise along with the latest knowledge on non-drug nutritional supplements. I was convinced that this solution would minimize the pain and progression of arthritis as well as dependence on medications and medical procedures, while enhancing mobility.

After I finished my worldwide travels, I created the Arthritis Rx Plan of exercise, diet, and supplements to treat the population afflicted with arthritis of the hip and knee, the most commonly affected joints. My exercise program uses the breath as an aid to pain control with safe exercises that minimize bad stresses to the arthritic joint. Your treatment goal, regardless of which of the one hundred types of arthritis you have, is to keep your pain under control. One way to do this is to focus on and regulate your breathing. Proper breathing in a slow, controlled rhythm is the fastest pain reliever you can use. It shifts the mind's attention away from the pain and the body's natural response to pain. We devote a portion of one chapter to thorough step-by-step instructions in deep breathing. In conjunction with proper breathing, my Arthritis Rx exercise regimen restores flexibility and strength, leading to less stress on the joint, reduction in pain, and enhancement of mobility.

Along with my colleagues Drs. Solomon, Adin, and Marrinan, I studied the effectiveness of this program in twenty-five patients with moderate knee and hip arthritis. This study, which has been presented at national academic meetings, will shortly be published in a peer-review journal. We studied nine men and sixteen women with a mean age of 52.3 years. The patients included in the study were still in pain despite using measures such as ice, heat, and oral medications consisting of anti-inflammatories and narcotics. All patients participated in the Arthritis Rx program three times per week for a period of one year. There was a 43 percent reduction in pain, a 46 percent reduction in anti-inflammatories taken, and a 50 percent reduction in narcotics taken at the end of one year. All the changes were statistically significant. My colleagues around the nation have done similar studies to show the effectiveness of proper exercise programs, including their role in decreasing pain and reliance on pain medications, as well as the potential impact on decreasing the progression of arthritis. I summarize their findings in this book.

My exercise regimen incorporates three key techniques for preventing and reducing the pain of arthritis: Pilates, yoga, and healthy breathing. Pilates exercises strengthen the core muscles of the body so that they work in harmony with the joints to provide a full range of movement. Yoga engages the entire body in healthy breathing while freeing the mind to focus without distraction or anxiety. Although proper forms of yoga and Pilates represent the best possible way to preserve joints, in the short run the vigorous twists, turns, and bends of advanced yoga can actually harm joints. *Arthritis Rx* overcomes this problem with a carefully sequenced instruction of yoga- and Pilates-based movements and postures that will strengthen the joints without harming them.

My exercise program contains three series of exercises to heal and strengthen your joints. Each series takes fifteen minutes to complete and should be done three times a week for a minimum of eight weeks. Series A alone will get you moving pain-free again after an acute joint injury. Many patients maintain good long-term joint health by continuing to do Series A regularly without moving on to Series B and C.

For those who want to raise their joint fitness for sports and recreational enjoyment or to ameliorate the effects of stress injury and age, Series B offers a vigorous routine. Series C provides a strenuous core body workout.

The vast majority of arthritis sufferers—more than 80 percent—can heal by following my exercise regimen and combining it with the use of heat and/or ice, along with the proper diet and judicious use of supplements. For the small percentage of people who need to take other measures as well, *Arthritis Rx* can be the foundation of an effective treatment program.

The experiences of people like my grandfather who successfully managed arthritis have transformed old assumptions. Studies have shown that the degree of damaged cartilage seen on X-rays is not a good predictor of the amount of pain and disability an individual with arthritis will encounter. Some people, like my grandfather, who have extensive damage and use exercise and other techniques to manage the condition, are minimally affected, whereas others who have moderate arthritis become disabled. Thanks to these findings, the medical community now considers multiple factors in coming up with a treatment plan, not just the degree of damaged cartilage on the X-ray.

Another change is that the principles of preserving the joints of professional athletes are now applied to people in every walk of life: those who have sedentary jobs that require them to sit in front of computer screens as well as those who have jobs that require them to be on their feet all day or to do a lot of bending and heavy lifting.

I have incorporated many of the techniques for treating pain that I learned as a consulting physician for the Association of Tennis Professionals (ATP) circuit and the Professional Golfer's Association (PGA) Tour. Treating professional athletes and their coaches has enabled me to observe how arthritis develops over the life span of an individual and what can be done at every stage to maintain the function of the joint.

Even though most professional athletes are in outstanding physical condition, they are prime candidates for arthritis. They overuse their joints and suffer recurring injuries. Hitting hundreds of balls each day or moving at breakneck speed on the tennis court takes its toll on the cartilage of hands, knees, and other joints. Athletes often don't remember specific injuries suffered during their playing days, but these injuries can accelerate cartilage destruction in their knees and hips, and can lead to pain and loss of mobility in later life.

My year on the road with the ATP tennis circuit showed me that no single therapy works for everyone afflicted by joint pain. Some players were helped by massage therapy, acupuncture, or chiropractic techniques. *Arthritis Rx* incorporates these insights and healing techniques from a wealth of perspectives. In Part Four, I provide suggestions for selecting the treatment appropriate to your individual needs.

Although this book focuses on arthritis of the knee and hip, the most common sites, the exercises and other information will also prove helpful for people with arthritis of the hands, shoulders, and other joints.

As the incidence of arthritis doubles over the next twenty-five years, minimally invasive, non-surgical therapies will play a strategic role in eliminating arthritis pain, enhancing mobility, and protecting cartilage. Future technologies will no doubt facilitate earlier diagnosis, so that early intervention can be initiated to retard the progression of arthritis. These "chondro-protective" therapies to safeguard the cartilage are so important that some experts have predicted that they will be as helpful to arthritis as penicillin was for the treatment of infectious diseases. I look forward to describing these approaches in greater detail at the end of this book.

Finally, no comprehensive arthritis program would be complete without a proper diet that, in conjunction with the Arthritis Rx exercise program, will keep your weight in check while reducing pain and enhancing mobility. Since finishing my Arthritis Rx exercise research, I have concentrated on putting together a proper diet and nutritional supplement for arthritis. The Arthritis Rx Diet is based on the concept of the anti-inflammatory diet. There is ample evidence that the standard American diet, which is very high in processed foods, contains tremendous amounts of processed sugars and saturated fats that promote not just obesity but also inflammation. Although osteoarthritis, which is the topic of this book, has traditionally been called non-inflammatory, there is evidence to show that it, too, has some level of inflammation. Inflammation is clearly linked to increase in loss of cartilage, leading to more arthritis as well as increase in heart disease, cancer, and diabetes. The data also show that people with severe inflammatory diseases such as rheumatoid arthritis are at very high risk for early heart disease. Chronic inflammation of the colon has been linked to colon cancer. Because these major public health issues share inflammation as a major causative factor, an anti-inflammatory diet such as the Arthritis Rx Diet is essential not only for a comprehensive treatment of arthritis but also for weight control and reduction of the chances of developing heart disease, cancer, and diabetes. My diet is based on clinical evidence of the food groups that can decrease inflammation and thereby reduce arthritis pain and the progression of the disease. The Arthritis Rx Diet also gives advice on the kinds of food to avoid, those that can lead to inflammation and more arthritic pain. I look forward to telling you more about the benefits of following the Arthritis Rx Diet in Chapter Five.

I have also helped in developing the Arthritis Rx nutritional supplement called Zingerflex (www.zingerflex.com). Each batch of this supplement is tested for purity by an independent evaluator (including companies such as Viosak, Inc., based in New York). The supplement is a combination of one of the oldest known natural anti-inflammatories, ginger, combined with glucosamine and chondroitin sulfate. Ginger and glucosamine have been studied extensively here as well as in Europe, with data published in prestigious American and European journals. Their role in diminishing arthritis pain with minimal side effects is well known. Two highly anticipated clinical trials whose results were released in November 2005 demonstrate emphatically the value of glucosamine and/or chondroitin in relieving pain in osteoarthritis patients. The multicentered Glucosamine/Chondroitin Arthritis Intervention Trial (GAIT) conducted by the National Institutes of Health involved more than 1,500 osteoarthritis patients who were given 1,500 mg/day of glucosamine hydrochloride and/or 1,200 mg/day chondroitin sulfate, as opposed to 200 mg/day of the common prescription pain medication celecoxib (Celebrex) or placebo for twenty-four weeks. The preliminary results indicate that both celecoxib and the glucosamine-chondroitin combination significantly reduced knee pain compared to the placebo, and that all treatments were well tolerated by the subjects. That is an extremely significant result, because glucosamine and chondroitin have no known side effects, compared to the well-documented dangers of COX-2 inhibitors such as Celebrex, including increased risk of high blood pressure and heart disease with prolonged use. These findings mean that glucosamine and chondroitin will now become the first-choice oral supplement that most doctors recommend to diminish arthritis symptoms. The GAIT results were bolstered by the preliminary results of another multicentered clinical study, the European-sponsored Glucosamine Unum in Die Efficacy (GUIDE) Trial, which compared the effect of 1,500 mg/day of glucosamine sulfate vs. 3,000 mg/day of acetaminophen or placebo over twenty-four weeks on various pain and mobility indices of osteoarthritis. The researchers reported that glucosamine sulfate was more effective than acetaminophen (Tylenol), and concluded that "glucosamine sulfate might be the preferred symptomatic medication in knee osteoarthritis," while reporting no differences in the relative safety of the two supplements. Both GAIT and the GUIDE trial are well-designed, well-conducted, "gold-standard" studies that conclusively prove the value of glucosamine and chondroitin in treating symptoms of osteoarthritis.

My supplement has the added pain-relief value of ginger, which has also been well-documented. Currently no other supplement on the market combines ginger with glucosamine and chondroitin sulfate. Apart from taking my supplement, it's easy to get more ginger into your diet, as I explain in Chapter Six.

The Arthritis Rx Plan is a holistic program born out of the influences of my life from early childhood and my medical training at a prestigious arthritis research institution, and further honed by my travels around the world as a visiting professor. I have been able to enhance and perfect the plan by having had the privilege of treating thousands of patients with arthritis. I strongly believe that this program will help anyone afflicted with arthritis at any stage of the disease process. *Arthritis Rx* is a comprehensive solution for eliminating arthritis pain, enhancing mobility, slowing the progression of arthritis, and restoring quality of life. The combination of the most advanced modern medicine with the ancient wisdom of yoga and the core strengthening of Pilates will empower you to take your healing into your own hands and become your own best healer.

# WHAT TO DO IF YOU ARE IN PAIN NOW

There is no cure for arthritis at the present time. *Arthritis Rx* is designed to help you manage arthritis without having to resort to surgery by minimizing the risk factors than can accelerate it and maximizing the factors that can slow its progression. We accomplish this by adopting an arthritis-friendly lifestyle of proper diet, supplements, and exercises. Your treatment goal, then, is to keep your pain under control. One way to do this is to focus on and regulate your breathing. Proper breathing in a slow, controlled rhythm is the fastest pain reliever you can use. It shifts the mind's attention away from the pain and the body's natural response to pain. If you are in pain now, the first thing to do is to try to relax. It's normal to tense up when in pain, so try to slow your breathing as much as possible and take full, deep breaths. If possible, inhale deeply through your nose and hold your breath in your lungs for a count of three. Exhale fully by contracting your stomach slightly, then inhale until you feel your stomach expanding somewhat. Continue breathing in this way for at least two to three minutes. Deep breathing not only delivers extra oxygen to overstressed muscles and disks, allowing them to begin to relax, but also calms the mind and nervous system and helps relieve pain. Repeat this process throughout the day whenever you feel pain or anxiety about your physical condition.

When you are in pain, you may also find visual imagery useful in guiding your breath and enhancing the relaxation response. For example, try imagining your breath as a wave of golden light flowing into the crown of your head and down through your spinal column. You may picture a thin hollow reed or tube stretching from the crown to the base of your spine, with the golden light descending the length of your spine and then spreading out to the rest of your body. Another good technique is to picture yourself in a favorite spot, real or imagined, where you feel safe and at ease. It could be a tree beside a quiet stream, a white sand beach, a mountain retreat, or just your backyard. The more relaxed your breathing becomes, the less pain you will feel. As you become better able to focus on your breathing for a few minutes at a time, you will also prepare your mind and body to work together on the rest of your healing. (I give much more detailed instructions on deep breathing in Chapter Three.)

Another good technique is to lie flat on the floor on your back with your knees up and your lower legs resting on a chair, an ottoman, or some pillows, or lie on your side in bed in the fetal position with a pillow between your knees. These positions should take the strain off your knees, hips, and lower back, but if another position feels better, that is fine. Let your body guide you into the least painful position possible.

In addition to proper breathing, here are some other steps to take if you are in pain right now:

## Medications

- Take anti-inflammatory and pain-relief medications to speed healing. Pain doesn't equal gain. Being overly stoic may actually slow your recovery. The most readily available over-the-counter pain relief medicines are aspirin, ibuprofen (Advil), acetaminophen (Tylenol), and naproxen (Aleve). Ibuprofen is generally the best choice for arthritis pain because it combines pain relief and anti-inflammatory benefits.
- Liquid gel pills work best; they are absorbed more readily in the bloodstream. As a general rule, unless a doctor prescribes otherwise, you should take two liquid gel ibuprofen two to three times a day.
- Everybody reacts to medicine slightly differently, and you may find that it helps to combine ibuprofen with acetaminophen, taking the first for pain and inflammation and the second for additional pain relief. In any case, do not take more than eight pills a day, total, unless your doctor prescribes otherwise.
- People with diabetes should be especially careful not to take high doses of anti-inflammatory medicines for extended periods because of the potential for kidney damage. Anti-inflammatory medications are also contraindicated

for those with a history of gastric ulcers or compromised kidney function. Patients who take Coumadin (warfarin), a blood thinner, should consult their physicians.

- If severe pain persists after seven to ten days of taking ibuprofen and/or acetaminophen, you should consult a physician.
- If over-the-counter medicines don't lessen your pain and inflammation significantly, don't wait an entire week to go to the doctor. More powerful pain relievers are available by prescription and are safe if used as directed.
- Like over-the-counter remedies, these medicines should be taken only short term. If they have not brought you any significant, lasting relief after a few days, you should consult your physician again.

### Water, Heat, Ice, and Liniments

- If you have access to a pool, aquatherapy can speed your recovery. Warm baths and showers can also be useful.
- In the first twenty-four to forty-eight hours after an injury to your knees or other joints, apply ice to tender areas two to three times a day for ten to fifteen minutes at a time, in order to lessen inflammation. Keeping the ice on longer won't give you any added benefit; it reaches its maximum efficacy after fifteen minutes.
- After forty-eight hours, apply moist heat in the shower or with a heating pad for up to thirty minutes at a time as desired. Unlike cold, gentle warmth may continue to provide an increased benefit if it is applied for a longer period of time.
- After forty-eight hours, use heat and ice in sequence. As a general rule, apply heat in the morning and before physical therapy or other activity, and apply ice after activity and in the evening at dinnertime or bedtime. Some people, however, get more relief from heat, whereas others get more from ice, so modify the sequence to fit your own needs.
- Apply liniments and rubs like Tiger Balm, Sportscreme, and BENGAY to soothe injured areas. The active ingredient in such products is usually

some form of rubbing alcohol, and they never penetrate below skin level. But the act of applying the rub, or having someone else do so for you, can itself be calming and beneficial from an emotional and psycho-physiological point of view.

- As the pain of your injury decreases, gradually increase your activity following the guidelines in Chapter Four.

# PART ONE

# WHAT IS ARTHRITIS,
# WHAT CAUSES IT,
# AND HOW
# CAN IT BE MANAGED?

# CHAPTER ONE

# HOW JOINTS WORK

The musculoskeletal system is a marvel of engineering that makes possible every imaginable movement of the human body. Think of a professional tennis player serving a ball at over one hundred miles per hour, a young gymnast doing a series of backflips, or a concert pianist's fingers playing hundreds of notes in a few seconds, bringing pleasure to thousands of people. The free and easy movement of childhood is a joy that we have all experienced. However, by the time we become adults, many of us find that pain has replaced pleasure as a result of arthritis, injuries, and overuse. Fortunately, if you have lost the joy of movement, you can almost always regain it.

Our increased understanding of how the elements of the musculoskeletal system work has resulted in a new standard of care for people suffering from arthritis: No longer is the goal merely to help patients regain movement. Today the gold standard is pain-free movement. Although the pain of arthritis and other barriers to movement can be intense, they can be overcome by following the pain-relief guidelines laid out in this book. Research has shown that the health of the musculo-skeletal system depends on the proper amount of exercise. If you do the exercises in this book for fifteen minutes three times a week, the odds of a recovery are over-whelmingly in your favor. Over 80 percent of the patients in my sports medicine practice have found lasting relief by following the exercise regimen. Adding to it an anti-inflammatory diet like the one I describe, and appropriate levels of nutritional supplements, will raise your chances of success even higher.

As its name implies, the musculoskeletal system consists of muscles (from the Latin word *musculus*) and bone (from the Greek word *skeletos*). Other key components include the joints (the junctions between two or more bones where movement takes place), the ligaments (fibrous bands of tissue that bind the parts of the joint together), and the tendons (fibrous cords that attach muscles to bones, stabilizing the joints as well as moving them). Like a delicate machine, all parts must be working properly to produce pain-free movement. Friction and injuries can set the stage for the development of arthritis, which can erode and destroy vital components of the network.

A total of 206 bones support the body. Although most people think of bones as solid, inert components, they are living tissues that are constantly being remodeled. Bones function as the body's depository for important minerals, such as calcium and phosphorus. These minerals keep bones strong so that they will be able to withstand the stress of movement. When you walk at a leisurely pace, each foot strikes the ground with a force about three times your weight. If you run, the pressure increases to five to six times.

The skeleton of the average person weighs about twenty pounds and is held together by over 650 muscles. The muscles perform double duty, lengthening and shortening to produce movement. Like bones, they are subject to stress. If you overstretch or overuse a muscle, pain results, as any weekend runner knows. More serious traumas can cause muscles to tear.

Together with the muscles and bones, the joints where bones meet play a key role in the musculoskeletal system. All joints have cartilage, a tough, somewhat elastic material that covers the ends of the bones, allowing them to glide across each other smoothly to produce movement. Cartilage acts like a cushion for the joint. Because it is about 75 percent water, cartilage compresses when pressure is applied and resumes its original thickness when force is withdrawn. But over time, friction harms the ability of cartilage to protect the bones. Scratches appear, and eventually the cartilage may be worn away. Bone then rubs on bone to produce arthritis.

Fortunately, the joints have an ally in the fight against friction: a liquid called synovial fluid that lubricates the joint like motor oil. The bursa is a small sac-shaped membrane filled with synovial fluid that is found in the knee and many other joints. The bursa acts like a cushion between the bone and the fibrous tissues of the muscles and tendons, making pain-free movement possible. Knees have an additional source of protection that enables them to withstand the shock of movement: the meniscus, the crescent-shaped cartilage located between the ends of the bone in the thigh and leg. However, certain impact injuries and twisting injuries, such as falling off a ladder or severely twisting your leg playing sports, can tear the meniscus, causing pain in the knee. A popping sound sometimes occurs at the moment of injury.

The labrum offers similar protection in the hip. The cartilage lines the socket (acetabulum) of the hipbone in which the ball of the thighbone (femur) sits. This cartilage also keeps the ball in the socket. A tear in the labral cartilage can cause pain or lead to arthritis.

Anatomical factors sometimes make joints vulnerable to injury and arthritis. Like door hinges, knees permit a wide range of motion: sliding, bending, gliding, and swiveling. They are in almost constant use and are subject to great friction. Although more stable than the knee, hips are also prime candidates for injuries and arthritis. The ball and socket joints of the hip must bear the weight of the body, which can also cause strain and damage cartilage.

The final element of the musculoskeletal system is the ligaments: tough, slightly elastic, fibrous bands that bind the bones together and help keep the joints in place. For example, those on either side of the knee joint prevent the bones from sliding out of joint.

Because all these elements have to work in tandem, if any one of them becomes damaged or malfunctions, it can compromise other elements in the system and lead to the development of arthritis, which I explain in the next chapter. When that occurs, the musculoskeletal system needs a recovery program that will give first aid to injured muscles and bones, improve the functioning of joints damaged by the loss of cartilage, and help us learn to listen to our bodies to enhance body awareness at every stage of life. The Arthritis Rx Plan treats arthritis in its earliest phases as well as its later stages. Its combination of rehabilitation exercises with medical adaptations of yoga and Pilates, proper diet, and supplements can help you enjoy pain-free movement every day.

Now let's look closely at what causes arthritis and what the Arthritis Rx Plan can do to preserve and enhance your mobility.

# CHAPTER TWO

# WHY ARTHRITIS DEVELOPS

$S$eptember 15 was a crucial day for John. The forty-seven-year-old entrepreneur was scheduled to present his business plan to a group of investors in hopes that they would fund an expansion of his retail business. That morning, however, John woke up with excruciating pain in his right knee. Thirty years of amateur soccer had taken its toll. He had been feeling some pain and soreness in the knee for several months, and had even been unable to play soccer for a time, but had blamed his condition on a collision he'd had on the field. He figured he would start playing again when the pain subsided. Now there was no getting around the fact that he could barely dress himself without experiencing severe pain and that he would have trouble driving to work.

Beverly, John's neighbor, also suffered pain that morning. The sixty-year-old teacher limped around her apartment. The pain in her left hip was so intense that she decided to call in sick. She had been experiencing the pain for several years, and as it continued to grow worse, she felt trapped by her increasing lack of mobility.

Both patients came to see me at the Hospital for Special Surgery, where my sports medicine practice is located. Like more than 66 million Americans, they were suffering from arthritis, one of the oldest and most chronic diseases in the world. Arthritis includes more than one hundred different disorders characterized by pain, swelling, and limited movement in the joints, from rheumatoid arthritis to osteoarthritis. John and Beverly have osteoarthritis, the most common form of arthritis. Osteoarthritis is caused by the breakdown and eventual loss of the cartilage in one or more joints. Because osteoarthritis is essentially a degenerative disease, it occurs more frequently and with greater severity as you age. It shows up more frequently in men over the age of forty-five and in women after age fifty-five, primarily from wear and tear on the joints. Other factors exacerbate osteoarthritis, including diet and weight, and some people who suffer from it have a genetic predisposition. Rheumatoid and psoriatic arthritis, which are primarily caused by severe inflammation within the joints that destroys the cartilage, are genetically transmitted. They are far less common than osteoarthritis.

The National Institute of Arthritis and Musculoskeletal and Skin Diseases (NIAMS) estimates that by 2030 about 70 million people—20 percent of the population—will be at risk for osteoarthritis because the disease becomes more common as people age. The 76 million baby boomers born between 1946 and 1964 are now entering middle age and are prime candidates to develop the disease. The loss of cartilage leads to the inflammation of the joints that is characteristic of osteoarthritis (Figure 1). The smooth layer of connective tissue that encases the ends of bones, cartilage enables bones to absorb the shock of joint motion, facilitating fluid, easy movement. Initially, the cartilage is able to repair itself, but over time the smooth surface breaks down and pieces float in the joint space. Bone spurs—sharp outcroppings—may develop at the edges of the bones that make up the joints and can cause further damage to the cartilage.

The progression of osteoarthritis varies from person to person. Some, like John, first notice pain and stiffness after engaging in a strenuous activity, such as his Saturday soccer matches. Others, like Beverly, experience daily pain that gradually gets

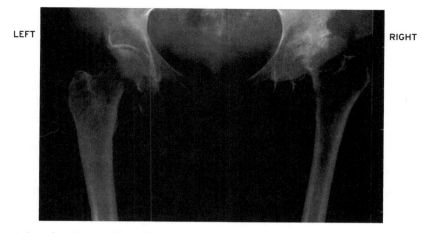

LEFT         RIGHT

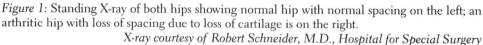

*Figure 1:* Standing X-ray of both hips showing normal hip with normal spacing on the left; an arthritic hip with loss of spacing due to loss of cartilage is on the right.

*X-ray courtesy of Robert Schneider, M.D., Hospital for Special Surgery*

worse. Although osteoarthritis is not life-threatening, it takes a severe toll on an individual's quality of life.

By age forty, about 90 percent of individuals have X-ray evidence of osteoarthritis in the weight-bearing joints such as the hips and knees. Some people aren't aware of the deterioration and feel little pain. Others, however, experience pain even when their joints are at rest. There is no predictable correlation between what we see on X-rays and the amount of pain or loss of motion a patient is experiencing. A person with very little arthritis on X-rays may have a lot of pain and vice versa. "My soccer game was my favorite activity of the week," said John. "When I couldn't participate, I felt depressed."

"Hip pain was shrinking my world," said Beverly. "At first, I would have only mild stiffness in the morning, but over the years the pain grew worse. I stopped dancing and doing my housework. I rarely stood in front of my classes, and missed many days of work."

Fortunately, I could reassure John and Beverly that, although there is no cure for osteoarthritis, if they follow the Arthritis Rx Plan, they will retain their mobility and continue to enjoy their normal activities. Physicians now know much more about who is likely to develop osteoarthritis. Here are the factors we have identified:

## HEREDITY

Like many conditions, osteoarthritis seems to run in families. One indication of a genetic predisposition is the appearance of Herberden's nodes. The hard, bony growths on the joints near the fingertips are twice as common in women whose mothers had these joint changes. Research is also underway to determine whether a mutation in a gene that affects the synthesis of type two collagen — the primary protein in cartilage — may play a role in the development of osteoarthritis.

## OBESITY

Obesity is another risk factor. Generally, the more a person weighs, the greater the pressure on the hips, knees, and other weight-bearing joints. Beverly, for example, had gained thirty pounds in the last twenty years. That's especially dangerous for women who want to avoid hip arthritis. The Nurses' Health Study — one of the largest studies of risk factors for chronic diseases in women — found that nurses who were overweight at age eighteen were five times more likely to develop hip arthritis in middle age than women who maintained a normal weight. This study has serious implications, because more than half of the women in the United States are overweight. Most men also weigh more than they should for optimal health. The hip joint, for example, experiences forces up to four times your body weight during walking. So if you are 30 pounds overweight, the hip is experiencing 120 pounds per square inch of extra force. The good news is that if you manage to lose even ten of those pounds, the hip will experience 40 pounds per square inch less force. This is one of the few times that you are guaranteed a 400 percent return on your investment. Lose one pound and take 4 pounds per square inch of force off your hip.

Weight management is a significant factor in the development of arthritis because excess poundage clearly creates a greater strain on the weight-bearing joints such as hips and knees. Being overweight or obese has become a national epidemic. The National Institutes of Health (NIH) reports that an estimated 60 percent of adult Americans are now overweight or obese. Even worse, the number of individuals who are obese has increased by more than one-third in the last twenty years. Children are also packing on the pounds: 10 percent of preschoolers were overweight in 2004.

These trends don't bode well for individuals who hope to avoid arthritis. Being overweight doesn't guarantee that you will develop arthritis, but it significantly increases your chances. A study by researchers at Boston University found that an obese woman could decrease her risk of developing arthritis of the knee by losing eleven pounds. The first step in determining a healthy weight is to figure out your body mass index (see chart on p. 28). In 1998 the NIH established the body mass index (BMI) because the formula, which considers the ratio of total body fat, is a more accurate measurement of health risks related to weight than the number on your bathroom scale or the old weight and height tables.

The experts who developed the guidelines determined that a BMI of 19 to 24 is desirable. They identified overweight as a BMI of 25 to 29.9 and obesity as a BMI of 30 and above. Extreme obesity is a BMI of 40 or higher. Studies show that individuals are at increased risk for development of arthritis, high blood pressure, and other related conditions if their BMI is 25 or greater. But BMI is not the only indicator of body fat, and you should use it in conjunction with common sense and a physician's recommendations. Because muscle weighs more than fat, a very muscular person might have a BMI of 30 and still be in good health. If you have a BMI of 25 or higher, however, you stand a good chance of being overweight and at risk for arthritis as well as other diseases.

To find your BMI, locate your height in the left column. Move across the chart until you find your approximate weight. Then follow that column down to the corresponding BMI number at the bottom of the chart.

| Height | | | | | | | | Body Weight in Pounds | | | | | | | |
|---|---|---|---|---|---|---|---|---|---|---|---|---|---|---|---|
| 4'10" | 91 | 96 | 100 | 105 | 110 | 115 | 119 | 124 | 129 | 134 | 138 | 143 | 148 | 153 |
| 4'11" | 94 | 99 | 104 | 109 | 114 | 119 | 124 | 128 | 133 | 138 | 143 | 148 | 153 | 158 |
| 5'0" | 97 | 102 | 107 | 112 | 118 | 123 | 128 | 133 | 138 | 143 | 148 | 153 | 158 | 163 |
| 5'1" | 100 | 106 | 111 | 116 | 122 | 127 | 132 | 137 | 143 | 148 | 153 | 158 | 164 | 169 |
| 5'2" | 104 | 109 | 115 | 120 | 126 | 131 | 136 | 142 | 147 | 153 | 158 | 164 | 169 | 174 |
| 5'3" | 107 | 113 | 118 | 124 | 130 | 135 | 141 | 146 | 152 | 158 | 163 | 169 | 175 | 180 |
| 5'4" | 110 | 116 | 122 | 128 | 134 | 140 | 145 | 151 | 157 | 163 | 169 | 174 | 180 | 186 |
| 5'5" | 114 | 120 | 126 | 132 | 138 | 144 | 150 | 156 | 162 | 168 | 174 | 180 | 186 | 192 |
| 5'6" | 118 | 124 | 130 | 136 | 142 | 148 | 155 | 161 | 167 | 173 | 179 | 186 | 192 | 198 |
| 5'7" | 121 | 127 | 134 | 140 | 146 | 153 | 159 | 166 | 172 | 178 | 185 | 191 | 197 | 204 |
| 5'8" | 125 | 131 | 138 | 144 | 151 | 158 | 164 | 171 | 177 | 184 | 190 | 197 | 203 | 210 |
| 5'9" | 128 | 135 | 142 | 149 | 155 | 162 | 169 | 176 | 182 | 189 | 196 | 203 | 209 | 216 |
| 5'10" | 132 | 139 | 146 | 153 | 160 | 167 | 174 | 181 | 188 | 195 | 202 | 207 | 215 | 222 |
| 5'11" | 136 | 143 | 150 | 157 | 165 | 172 | 179 | 186 | 193 | 200 | 208 | 215 | 222 | 229 |
| 6'0" | 140 | 147 | 154 | 162 | 169 | 177 | 184 | 191 | 199 | 206 | 213 | 221 | 228 | 235 |
| BMI | 19 | 20 | 21 | 22 | 23 | 24 | 25 | 26 | 27 | 28 | 29 | 30 | 31 | 32 |

## TRAUMA

Often a severe trauma such as a motor vehicle accident or fall may cause damage to the cartilage. Many times it may take more than a year for arthritis to develop in the joint that was traumatized. Even a small tear in the cartilage can lead to inflammation at the site of the injury. If that inflammation remains unchecked for more than a short time, it can lead to significant damage to the cartilage. This injury can be the instigating factor that leads to loss of resiliency in the cartilage, earlier cartilage breakdown, and thus arthritis.

## AGING

Until the 1980s many patients like Beverly considered osteoarthritis a natural occurrence of aging. Although the condition becomes increasingly common in the forties, fifties, and sixties, aging per se isn't responsible. Research has shown that there are several differences between an aging joint and one affected by osteoarthritis. Osteoarthritis causes changes in the bone below cartilage that don't occur in an aging joint. Although cartilage loses water content with aging, it can lose that water content more rapidly in an arthritic joint. Changes in the bone below the arthritic joint may also contribute to further cartilage deterioration. Some of the newer research is aimed at preserving the bone right below the cartilage.

## ESTROGEN

The hormone estrogen may also play a role in the development of osteoarthritis in women. After menopause, the amount of estrogen in the body plummets. Several studies have found that estrogen replacement therapy may have a protective effect on bone in older women. However, when estrogen replacement therapy is stopped, the benefits decline. Within ten years, risk gradually returns to a level similar to that of women who have never used estrogen replacement therapy.

I advise my female patients to carefully review their decisions to take estrogen replacement therapy with their primary care doctor. Recent studies have found that estrogen replacement therapy has a downside: increased risks for breast cancer, heart attacks, and strokes, so women must weigh advantages and disadvantages carefully. Nonetheless, there is enough evidence to show that higher estrogen levels have a cartilage-protective effect. I have seen many women in my practice who have accelerating arthritis with loss of cartilage after menopause. Each woman must consider the risk and benefits of hormone replacement individually with her physician to see if it is right for her.

## CALCIUM AND VITAMIN D

Scientists are studying whether diet plays a role in the onset of arthritis. Calcium is the main component of bone, and vitamin D is necessary for calcium absorption. Diets low in calcium and vitamin D accelerate the development of osteoporosis, a condition that leads to fragile bones and fractures. Studies are underway to determine whether the lack of this mineral and vitamin affect the development of osteoarthritis too, because one of the pre-arthritic events involves softening of the bone immediately underneath the cartilage.

## OCCUPATION

We know much more today about the role of occupational factors in developing arthritis. Heavy physical labor may damage the joints and set the stage for osteoarthritis. For example, dockworkers, miners, and furniture movers often develop osteoarthritis in their knees. Fortunately, there are ways to modify jobs to prevent damage to joints by overuse. Physical therapists have developed programs to teach proper body mechanics for manual labor when arthritis is present in a particular joint. Employers may also be willing to modify job descriptions or workplace environments to include some deskwork or to minimize heavy lifting, squatting, or climbing stairs. One of my patients, whom I'll call Jim, is forty-two years old and has knee arthritis. Because his work involved significant amounts of squatting and lifting heavy weights eight to ten hours per day, part of his treatment involved work modification, which we organized with his employer. Together we convinced his employer to change Jim's workload so that he is now doing four hours of heavy manual labor that prevents his having to squat at all, combined with four hours of paperwork. This has enabled Jim to continue to work while maintaining a relatively pain-free and mobile knee joint. It also made economic sense for his employer because the company has been able to avoid having Jim out for an extended period for surgery or on disability altogether.

## OTHER CONDITIONS

A range of other conditions may lead to osteoarthritis, especially in young adults. Individuals who suffer from metabolic disorders such as hemochromatosis (an inherited condition that causes the body to absorb and store too much iron, eventually damaging internal organs) and ochronosis (a blue-black discoloration of connective tissue including bone, cartilage, and skin caused by deposits of ochre-colored pigment) may develop osteoarthritis in their twenties and thirties. Musculoskeletal and connective tissue disorders such as Legg-Calve Perthes disease and hypermobility disorders such as Ehlers-Danlos Syndrome may lead to early osteoarthritis. These conditions interfere with proper metabolism of the cartilage, which leads in turn to early cartilage loss in individuals affected by these types of disorders. I recommend aquatherapy for patients with these disorders because water takes the stress off the joints while keeping strength intact. You can contact the Arthritis Foundation (see Appendix) for the aquatherapy program for arthritis nearest you.

## SPORTS INJURIES

Injuries suffered in contact sports often lead to osteoarthritis. Ten years ago, for example, during a soccer game John tore his meniscus, the wedgelike rubbery cushion where the bones of the leg connect. Meniscus tears are serious. In addition to helping the knee joint carry weight, glide, and turn in many directions, the meniscus keeps the thighbone and shinbone from grinding against each other. John didn't realize he had suffered these injuries and kept playing anyway. Several days later he developed severe pain and was treated for the injury. Like many athletes who suffer meniscus tears, fractures, and ligament injuries, John went on to develop arthritis of the knee.

I treat many athletes who play contact sports such as football, lacrosse, soccer, and rugby, and who in their early forties have developed significant knee arthritis as a result of repeated trauma and early cartilage wear. These sports involve significant shear stresses—uneven stresses to the cartilage that occur during activities such as rapid change in direction. Excessive shear stresses have been shown to lead to cartilage loss.

Ample evidence exists that non-contact sports such as golf and tennis can lead to arthritis of the lead hip. Having had close contact with the PGA Tour and the professional men's tennis circuit, I conducted research trials on both of these groups of professional athletes, and my findings were published in the *American Journal of Sports Medicine* in 2004. I was amazed at how many similarities I found between athletes of both sports in their lead hip. (If you are right-handed, then the left hip is your lead hip.) Forty-four percent of professional golfers and 40 percent of professional tennis players had significantly decreased flexibility of the lead hip that led to back pain. The repeated pivoting on the lead hip creates contractures in the capsule, the sac that surrounds the lead hip. These contractures lead to loss of flexibility. There is a clear connection between excessive loss of flexibility and eventual development of lead hip arthritis as these athletes age. The good news for all amateur tennis players and golfers is that by using the knowledge we have gained from studying the professionals, amateurs can minimize the chances of developing lead hip arthritis by following exercise programs such as Arthritis Rx.


## COMING UP WITH A DIAGNOSIS


When a patient like John comes to me complaining of joint pain and stiffness, I do what physicians have traditionally done: I take a complete, extensive medical history and make a thorough physical examination. This process, which we refer to as "history and physical," is the basic diagnostic tool for all physicians, and in the case of potentially arthritis-induced pain, is more helpful than all the X-rays and MRIs in the world. When I am trying to determine whether a patient who comes to me has arthritis, I look for two main criteria. Does he or she have pain that increases with activity? And is that pain accompanied by a loss in range of motion? Many people have old aches and pains, or recent physical impairments of many kinds that cause them pain, but that doesn't automatically mean that they have arthritis. Sharp pains in the elbow or knee could be the result of an injury, or they could be symptomatic of some larger illness. Only a detailed medical history and a hands-on physical examination can help the physician determine whether the pain the patient is reporting comes from arthritis or from some other source. Pain in the knee, for example, could be the result of a tearing of the meniscus, the cushion within the knee that helps the joint move fluidly. The patient will often report clicking, catching, or snapping sensations when trying to walk or bend. But the cause may be a sports-related incident, or something as common as slipping on the ice or getting out of a car, and may not be the result of arthritis at all.

The physical exam includes inspection of all joints in the hands, arms, legs, and feet. One of the first symptoms I look for when I palpate the joint (feel it with my hand) is jointline tenderness. The jointline is the place where the bones of the joint meet; in the knee, for instance, it's the line where the femur (thighbone) and tibia (shinbone) meet beneath the kneecap (patella). Tenderness to the touch along the jointline is a good indication of pathology, but once again the cause could be a recent injury of some kind. To be indicative of arthritis, the pain must be persistent, must be present over a long period of time (more than just a few weeks), and must get worse with activity. If you find that you can no longer bend over and tie your shoelaces as you once could, or have increasing difficulty making it up a flight of stairs, those are good indications that you may have arthritis. But only a doctor can determine this for certain.

If the cause of the pain and loss of motion remains unclear after taking your medical history and performing a complete physical examination, the physician may rely on other tests. You may need to get a blood analysis to rule out other autoimmune diseases. Or your doctor may request X-rays if she deems it necessary. But

X-rays are not foolproof because they often fail to detect small amounts of incipient damage. Magnetic resonance imaging, or MRI, is a more thoroughly predictive procedure but is also much more expensive—as much as $1,500—and so should be used only in cases when it is impossible to be certain through other tests. In an MRI we look for cartilage sequences—specific images that show the cartilage in detail and allow the physician to see very small amounts of cartilage deterioration. The Hospital for Special Surgery has developed a highly regarded procedure for giving and interpreting MRIs to detect cartilage damage. The vast majority of patients who complain of pain and loss of motion, however, can be diagnosed without resorting to radiology or blood work. History combined with physical examination remains the most important way to diagnose arthritic ailments.

I also want to know what, if anything, brings relief. I ask if pain gets better with rest or if stiffness improves with exercise. We discuss at length how symptoms have affected work and personal lives. Can they participate in sports? Is it painful to go up and down stairs? If a patient reports chronic pain in the knee from climbing stairs, or pain in the groin after walking long distances, these may be indicative of knee or hip arthritis. I also ask questions about skin, heart, lungs, and eyes because these organs can be involved in other types of arthritis. Excessive morning stiffness may also indicate other forms of arthritis, such as rheumatoid or psoriatic arthritis. These are essentially autoimmune disorders not caused by wear and tear, as osteoarthritis is.

Rheumatoid arthritis is a chronic, inflammatory form of the disease that affects not only cartilage and bone but other tissues and organs throughout the body as well. Although scientists don't know why rheumatoid arthritis develops, they suspect that an unidentified virus stimulates the immune system. As a result, the disease-fighting cells inflame the joints. Multiple joints are usually involved, especially on both sides of the body. Rheumatoid arthritis is a systemic disease: It can harm the heart, lungs, blood vessels, eyes, lymph nodes, and spleen. Common symptoms include fatigue, fever, and weakness. The condition waxes and wanes, and is not as persistent as osteoarthritis.

Psoriatic arthritis is another form of inflammatory arthritis. About one in ten individuals with psoriasis—a common skin disorder in which the skin becomes red and inflamed—may develop some pain and discomfort in affected joints, especially in those of the fingers and feet. Fortunately, psoriatic and many other forms of arthritis are quite rare, but those who have them can benefit from the regimens of my Arthritis Rx Plan. In this book, however, we concentrate on the more common osteoarthritis. In the next chapter, we look at the benefits of various exercises. For brevity, we will use the term arthritis rather than osteoarthritis.

# CHAPTER THREE

# THREE KEYS TO SLOWING THE PROGRESSION OF ARTHRITIS: FLEXIBILITY, STRENGTH, AND ENDURANCE

Despite what you may have been told, and contrary to the titles of several books on the subject, there is no cure for arthritis at the present time. It's a chronic disease similar in many ways to diabetes, cancer, and heart disease. Even something as drastic as knee replacement surgery amounts to little more than amputating the joint and replacing it with metal or ceramic. Surgery is not a cure—it's just another way of managing the disease. But although you can never entirely cure arthritis, you can learn to manage the pain and slow its progression. The Arthritis Rx Plan is designed to help you live with arthritis pain-free, without having to resort to surgery. The key to success in eliminating arthritis pain is to minimize the risk factors than can accelerate arthritis and maximize the factors that can slow its progression. We accomplish this by adopting an arthritis-friendly lifestyle of proper diet, supplements, and exercise.

Arthritis has been called the sneak thief of mobility and for good reason. As cartilage is worn away over several years, a cascade of changes takes place in the musculoskeletal system that gradually robs individuals of flexibility, strength, and endurance. This gradual destruction of cartilage sets in motion a disabling downward spiral. Movement becomes painful, so people become less active, and this in turn makes it even more difficult to remain mobile. Activities once enjoyed, such as cycling or biking, become impossible. Eventually, some individuals can't even perform simple movements such as opening a jar or walking up stairs. According to Kenneth Brandt, M.D., professor and head of the Rheumatology Division at the Indiana University School of Medicine, "Knee arthritis is the major cause of chronic disability in older people. Not fingers, not back, but knee. The pain of arthritis is typically made worse when you're weight-bearing and relieved by rest, so if you stand up and your knee hurts, you become a couch potato."

But the good news is that individuals can reverse this disabling cascade of cartilage changes with an exercise program like the one I prescribe that emphasizes three interrelated components of musculoskeletal health: flexibility, strength, and endurance.

- Flexibility is the ability to absorb and channel forces within the body, to bend without breaking.
- Strength is the ability to exert force.
- Endurance is the ability to do things again and again without tiring.

All of these factors are involved in movement. Flexibility forms the basis for strength and endurance, which in turn affect balance. Loss of balance is dangerous for those with arthritis; it can lead to falls and fractures.

Flexibility is the first casualty in the downward cascade. Flexibility is extremely important for the health of joints because it enables them to move as far as possible in every direction without pain. Some joints like the fingers are designed to bend and straighten. Others like those in the wrist can not only bend and straighten but also move away from and toward the middle of the body. The hips and shoulders are the most versatile joints in the body. They move in all three planes: flexing and bending, moving away from and toward the midline of the body, and rotating.

Arthritis robs joints of their range of motion. As arthritis proceeds, the normally smooth cartilage roughens, causing pitting, distortions, and eventually breakage. Joints can move fewer and fewer degrees, making familiar movements difficult. Typists find that their fingers can't perform certain strokes on their computer keyboards. Individuals who knit end up with stiff wrists when they practice their craft. For some people, the loss of motion is so great that they can't even put on their shoes.

The loss of motion causes pain, which accelerates the disabling cascade of changes in the musculoskeletal system. To protect their painful joints, many people minimize their movements. This harms the muscles as well as the joints because muscles that are not exercised weaken quickly, diminishing their ability to support joints properly. As a result, the range of motion becomes even more limited and muscles shut down.

Strong muscles are crucial both for preventing the onset of arthritis and for reducing its symptoms. As people get older, muscle mass declines. After age forty, muscle mass decreases about 1 percent a year. As a result, the average seventy-year-old has lost 30 percent of the muscle mass and strength he or she had at forty. Weak muscles make it difficult to balance the body properly when moving or even standing still or to catch yourself if you trip, and they also lead to early fatigue. Minor exertions such as carrying groceries become difficult. Consequently, work and personal lives suffer. Dr. Brandt has been at the cutting edge of research into the relationship between arthritis, muscle strength, and exercise. His most recent study, still unpublished, suggests that weakness in the quadriceps, a group of four muscles along the front of the thigh, may be a risk factor for arthritis. "Certainly quadriceps weakness can be the result of painful arthritis," Dr. Brandt says. "It's common to see quadriceps muscle weakness in people who have chronic arthritis, or chronic knee pain, regardless of the cause. As a result [of] disuse . . . the muscles shrink and atrophy. There's no question about that. But the newer concept is that weakness of the quadriceps may not only be the result of painful arthritis, but may actually be a cause of knee arthritis."

If he's correct, and I believe he is, then exercise can not only help to slow the progression of arthritis but may also prevent its onset in the first place. Indeed, current research shows that sound exercise programs like Arthritis Rx can help reverse this harmful cascade of changes that lead to a loss of joint flexibility and muscle strength. "There is some data to suggest that proper strengthening of the quadriceps may slow the rate of joint space narrowing," Dr. Brandt adds. "Certainly there are a number of studies in patients who have painful arthritis to show that strengthening the quads may decrease the joint pain." However, patients must be careful to avoid improper forms of quadriceps strengthening, such as using the knee-extension machine in most gyms, which has recently been shown to increase pain and potentially accelerate arthritis in the knee. Therefore, this particular type of quadriceps-strengthening exercise should be avoided.

My Arthritis Rx Exercise Series A focuses mostly on flexibility. It restores range of motion by putting sustained stress on the joint capsule, which helps the cartilage regain its elasticity without further harming the joint. By emphasizing exercises derived from physical therapy, Series A lays the foundation of core muscle flexibility and builds the strength needed for daily tasks and recreation. By focusing on muscles that are used to walk up stairs or rise from a chair, the exercises enable many people to regain their abilities to perform daily tasks.

With renewed flexibility, individuals with arthritis are able to use Series B to reverse the second casualty of the downward cascade—the loss of strength. Series B emphasizes the development of muscle strength with yoga-based work that intensifies the loading of core muscles. Later individuals can use Series C to further maximize joint mobility and strength training to maximize endurance.

## YOGA AND PILATES

As I mentioned earlier, although full-scale yoga and Pilates are the most effective methods for maximizing joint health, they both contain positions and movements that can easily traumatize a weak joint. The yoga- and Pilates-based elements of Arthritis Rx have been modified to eliminate these extreme stresses. What remains is a hallmark of both yoga and Pilates, the combination of targeted muscle work with proper breath control. The ancient yogis were the first to note the link between mind and breath. When we are agitated, our breathing accelerates and becomes shallower. When we are calm, our breathing slows and deepens. Using this principle, the various yoga postures for meditation and physical development have evolved to facilitate improved breathing so that every cell of the body benefits.

Modern scientific studies have shown that yoga is effective because its postures and controlled breathing provide high levels of oxygen to nourish muscles, ligaments, tendons, and other tissues. Joseph Pilates (1880–1967), founder of the Pilates exercises, also capitalized on the principles of yoga. He regularly took yoga postures and their carefully controlled breathing as a starting point, and then added dynamic muscle work to accelerate each posture's ability to enhance flexibility, strength, and endurance.


## DEEP BREATHING

Hatha (pronounced HUH-tuh) yoga, the physical training that is yoga's most familiar face in the Western world, helped establish the practice of forceful breathing. We take approximately 21,600 breaths in the course of a day. Most of the time we take short, shallow "rabbit" breaths into the upper part of the lungs. This kind of breathing activates the sympathetic stress receptors that predominate there and are designed to function in emergencies. Activating these receptors triggers increases in heart rate, constricts the blood vessels so circulation becomes more efficient, and heightens blood pressure. These are all parts of an evolutionary survival mechanism designed to get us through a crisis—to escape danger or engage in combat, the "fight or flight" response. At the same time, however, the body releases stress-fighting hormones and produces harmful free radicals, hikes the levels of insulin and cholesterol, and stops burning fat for fuel (in case we need it later). These are all helpful in a momentary crisis when quick, intensive action is required. But if this behavior persists over a long period, it is ultimately destructive and life-shortening rather than life-preserving.

How you breathe will also determine whether your body stores or burns fat. Contrary to conventional wisdom, if you push yourself too hard when exercising, to the point where you are gasping for air and are forced to take shallow breaths, you will not burn fat and lose weight at all. If, on the other hand, you learn to breathe deeply into the lungs, you will activate the calming receptors located in the lower lobes. Not only will you feel more relaxed, but your body will also perceive that it is all right to burn its emergency stores of fat. The calming effects of deep breathing have been well known for thousands of years in the East, from the yogis of India to the Zen monks of Japan. But over the last century, the process has been passed to the West and is fairly easy to learn. The key is to motivate yourself to do it regularly. Here are the basic steps.

1. Sit in a chair with both feet flat on the floor, legs uncrossed. If you are comfortable sitting on a meditation cushion with legs crossed, by all means do so, but it isn't essential.

2. Close your mouth. Place one hand on your stomach around the navel to help you feel the action of your breath as it enters and leaves the stomach area. Breathe deeply through your nose into the stomach until you can feel your stomach expanding. Hold the breath for a moment.

3. Then exhale through your nose, consciously contracting your stomach until you've expelled as much air as you can. (Avoid straining to suck in the stomach, however.) Hold that emptiness for a moment before inhaling again. Once you have learned to expand and contract the belly, you can remove your hand and place both palms on your thighs, just behind the knee, or fold them in your lap.

4. The body's natural energy has an electrical component, and it can be charged more efficiently when you complete the circuit while breathing. To do this when you inhale, place the tip of your tongue against the soft palate at the top of your mouth, about midway between the teeth and the uvula or throat.

5. As you exhale, curl the tongue downward to contact the soft membrane that lies beneath it.

**6.** Repeat the cycle of breathing for at least five minutes at a time. As you progress, allow the breaths to gradually grow deeper and slower.

**As with any exercise program, ask your physician whether you should start the Arthritis Rx Plan. This is especially important if you have a heart condition, diabetes, high blood pressure, or any other medical problem that has an impact on your health.** Once you get the go-ahead from your physician, feel free to move through the sequences of the A, B, and C series at your own pace. But don't jump ahead. You should not attempt Series B until you can do Series A totally pain-free, and you should not attempt Series C—or full-scale yoga or Pilates—until you can do Series B totally pain-free.

Please keep in mind, however, that you can complete the Arthritis Rx program and restore mobility simply by doing Series A, which is designed to get you moving again without pain. Arthritis is a chronic condition, and so you should follow this plan throughout life for best results. Many people maintain joint health by doing Series A consistently. Those who want to reach substantially higher levels of joint mobility and flexibility progress to Series B and C.

You may have some mild pain during the first two to three weeks of doing the Arthritis Rx exercises. As flexibility increases, the pain will subside during the fourth to fifth weeks. By eight weeks, you will feel the therapeutic benefits of doing the exercises, since you have reversed the downward spiral, making better balance and endurance possible. You should follow the exercises a minimum of three times each week thereafter.

No matter what series you reach, keep in mind that pain does not equal gain. If you experience sharp pain at any time, first take a break and then try to do the movement more precisely and gently. You should expect and tolerate a little discomfort as you press to the limit of your stretch, but not more than that. If sharp pain persists no matter how gingerly you try to do the movement, you should stop and consult a physician.

Naturally, it's more fun to resume some of your favorite exercise and sports activities while following the Arthritis Rx exercise regimen. If you tell patients who have painful knees that they have to exercise, they get put off. But several studies show that patients can increase aerobic fitness with activities that don't increase their pain or their need for pain medication. Exercise is a pejorative word to most people. Activity is probably a better term. But the fact is, exercise or physical activity is like a drug in improving pain, like another pain pill.

Best of all, it's a pill that doesn't have negative side effects when taken properly. The Framingham Osteoarthritis Study was based in part on a segment of the famous Framingham Heart Study that was assessed in the early 1980s, at which time patients had been observed for over thirty-five years and many risk factors for osteoarthritis had been ascertained. Among its results was evidence that there was a direct link, especially in women, between being overweight and the risk of knee arthritis. Women who were in the top 20 percent of the population for body weight had about seven times the risk of developing knee arthritis compared with normal-weight women. So staying active to keep your weight down is essential. Just be careful what you do. Consult the following list to determine which forms of activity are safe and which are risky.

| ARTHRITIS-FRIENDLY ACTIVITIES | | ACTIVITIES TO AVOID |
|---|---|---|
| *Safe* | *Moderate* | *Unsafe* |
| Arthritis Rx exercises | Golf | Jogging, running |
| Aquatherapy | Cross-country skiing | Stairmaster |
| Swimming | Softball | Football |
| Walking briskly | Elliptical trainer | Soccer |
| Bicycling | Gardening (with stool) | Basketball |
| Low-impact aerobics | Tennis | Hockey |
| | Yoga, Pilates | Rock climbing |

## CHOOSING THE RIGHT HEALTH-CARE PRACTITIONER

Many people with arthritis can follow my Arthritis Rx Plan on their own, but others find it useful to have a physician's guidance and support. Family practice doctors and internists who provide primary care are well qualified to diagnose arthritis; coordinate the treatments of specialist physicians, physical therapists, and other caregivers; and provide suggestions and support for maintaining optimal joint health. During Stage One care, they can provide suggestions and encouragement to stick with Arthritis Rx or a similar program long enough for complete healing to occur.

The specialist physicians most often involved in arthritis treatment include rheumatologists, orthopedic surgeons, and physiatrists. Except for physiatrists, specialists generally do not participate in Stage One care. In later stages of care, a rheumatologist can be helpful if the patient needs oral medications (NSAIDs or COX-2 inhibitors) or if multiple joints are involved. Rheumatologists can help rule out other forms of arthritis, especially if the patient has morning stiffness.

Orthopedic surgeons can help you decide if surgical intervention will reduce your severe pain and restore function. They also can advise you on whether you are a suitable candidate for total joint replacement and other treatments.

Physiatrists have an important role to play in every stage of arthritis. As primary care physicians for the musculoskeletal system and specialists in physical medicine and rehabilitation, physiatrists have completed extensive training in conservative, non-surgical care for arthritis. Some physiatrists have also completed fellowships in spine and sports medicine, which can be useful in Stages Two to Four. They can recommend minimally invasive, non-surgical treatments that will enable patients to decrease pain and improve function.

All things considered, when faced with arthritis pain, most people turn first to their present primary care physician and his or her referral network. A physician who is aware of your medical and family history, has treated you for other conditions, and has earned your trust and confidence has a better chance of getting your recovery launched. Primary care physicians who have worked with you over the years also know what it takes to keep you on track better than a physician you have never worked with before.

If you don't have a personal physician or need a specialist, ask friends, family, and other people you trust and respect for recommendations. Professional organizations such as the American Academy of Orthopaedic Surgeons (aaos.org), the American Academy of Physical Medicine and Rehabilitation (aapmr.org), the American College of Rheumatology (rheumatology.org), and other groups listed throughout this book provide information about their specialists. They also have lists of practitioners who have completed advanced training and passed qualifying examinations. These lists can be helpful if you have recently moved.

In addition to general practice and specialist MDs, a number of other caregivers treat arthritis, including physical therapists, osteopaths, massage therapists, chiropractors, and acupuncturists. Whereas MDs and physical therapists are said to practice conventional medicine, the other caregivers are said to provide complementary treatments that ease pain and improve the quality of life, although, as I explain later, I prefer the term "integrative." A major difference between conventional and integrative medicine is that the effectiveness and safety of techniques used in conventional medicine have been verified in well-designed scientific studies. In the past, there have been few clinical trials of the techniques used in integrative medicine, but that is now beginning to change. The National Institutes of Health (NIH)—the federal government's medical research arm—have established a National Center for Complementary and Alternative Medicine that funds and conducts scientific studies. Of the common alternatives to conventional medical care for arthritis, only massage therapy and acupuncture have so far been proven effective in clinical trials. There is other, if less rigorous, medical evidence of the value of osteopathic and chiropractic care, however, and I have seen many patients helped by each of them.

Often the best way to find a practitioner is to ask others who have worked with the practitioners. You may also want to meet with the caregiver and ask about his or her training, methods, and philosophy of care. Be sure to tell the practitioner how arthritis impacts your life, and suggest that he or she discuss your treatment with your primary physician, who is managing your overall care.

Finally, use common sense. A friend or co-worker may have benefited from a particular technique, but that technique might not do anything for you. Every patient's arthritis is different. If a particular complementary technique doesn't help you over the course of several months, you should discontinue it and explore other therapies that may be better suited to your arthritis symptoms and lifestyle.

More information about these various treatment options can be found in Part Four.

PART TWO

# THE ARTHRITIS
# Rx PLAN

# CHAPTER FOUR

# STAGE ONE CARE: THE ARTHRITIS Rx PLAN

The first directive in the Hippocratic oath that all physicians take is to do no harm. I take that seriously when I set about treating patients whom I have diagnosed with arthritis. I would like to refrain from medical intervention to the greatest extent possible. I realize that this isn't always possible; some patients have waited too long to seek treatment, and are already at the stage when some form of invasive procedure may be required to relieve their pain and return them to full mobility. But at whatever stage of the disease they come to me, I begin by laying out the range of possible treatments, and the assurance that I will take the least invasive path to helping them heal.

Treatments for arthritis fall into four main categories, or stages. The vast majority of patients will achieve full mobility with Stage One care. The rest will benefit by combining Stage One care with Stage Two, Three, or Four. Stage One care consists of the comprehensive Arthritis Rx Plan that forms the core of this book. It comprises lifestyle modification with proper exercise, diet, and nutritional supplements to manage arthritis without involving the intervention of specialized health-care practitioners, although I do recommend consulting with your primary care physician before starting.

Stage Two care involves supplementing the Arthritis Rx Plan of Stage One with conventional oral medications and/or a wide range of integrative practitioners, without resorting to physically invasive procedures. Stage Three care makes use of minimally invasive, non-surgical procedures, such as hylan or cortisone injections, also accompanied by the Arthritis Rx Plan. And Stage Four encompasses a variety of invasive surgical procedures. In this chapter we look at the Arthritis Rx Plan that constitutes Stage One care before moving on to the other stages in subsequent chapters.

The first and most important step in treating your arthritis pain is to visit a medical doctor to determine that the pain and loss of mobility you are experiencing are actually caused by arthritis. There are other diseases or ailments that can cause pain and loss of mobility, including autoimmune diseases and neuromuscular diseases. If you have a family doctor or primary care physician who is familiar with your medical history, that's the person to talk to first about your concerns. If not, you should try to see a local physician who has been recommended by friends, family members, or co-workers. Once a physician has diagnosed you and determined that your symptoms reflect the onset of arthritis, you should immediately begin the Arthritis Rx Plan.


## THE PLAN


Almost everyone with arthritis can benefit from Stage One care. The advantage of this Arthritis Rx Plan is that you can follow it on your own without the need for further help from medical personnel. It is a three-pronged approach to enhancing joint health that emphasizes a healthy lifestyle and consists of:

1. The Arthritis Rx Diet, an anti-inflammatory diet regimen based on the latest research in using the right foods to combat inflammation

2. The use of the Arthritis Rx nutritional supplement called Zingerflex and other supplements that have been proven in clinical studies to have a powerful anti-inflammatory and cartilage-protective effect

3. A step-by-step Arthritis Rx exercise plan that has been shown in our own studies to diminish pain, enhance mobility, slow the progression of arthritis, and decrease the need for pain medications

As the Arthritis Rx Diet shows, it is essential to eat anti-inflammatory foods such as fish, vegetables, and fruits, which are thought to decrease inflammation, while eliminating foods loaded with refined sugars, processed foods, red meat, carbonated drinks, and other foods that are high in calories and cause more inflammation. Chapter Five presents the Arthritis Rx Diet in detail and explains what causes inflammation, how it can result in chronic arthritis (as well as a host of other chronic illnesses), and how to combat it.

Nutritional supplements such as glucosamine, chondroitin sulfate, and ginger may also be added to Stage One care, as recent studies have shown their value for arthritis sufferers. A study done at the University of Miami in 2001, and published in *Arthritis & Rheumatism*, for example, showed that 510 mg of ginger extract had statistically significant effects on relieving symptoms of knee arthritis. There were few side effects, the worst being mild stomach irritation. And a study by Dr. J. Y. Reginster, published in the prestigious British journal *The Lancet* in 2001, showed that 1,500 mg of glucosamine had a statistically significant effect on reducing symptoms of knee arthritis. No adverse side effects were reported. Zingerflex, the Arthritis Rx nutritional supplement that I have created, is composed of glucosamine, chondroitin sulfate, and ginger. (Find more about it at zingerflex.com or amazon.com.) Taking it in the amounts I recommend enhances the effects of the Arthritis Rx Plan by helping to decrease pain and inflammation while increasing mobility. I go into more depth about the proper supplements to decrease the pain of arthritis in Chapter Six.

If you are overweight, weight loss is imperative, since extra pounds strain your joints, add to your pain, and accelerate the progression of arthritis. So, in addition to proper diet and nutritional supplements, exercise is crucial. Water exercises (aquatherapy) and other aerobic activity should be used in conjunction with the Arthritis Rx exercise program to maintain aerobic fitness. (Contact the Arthritis Foundation, arthritis.org, to find the aquatherapy center nearest you.) Do the aerobic activity that gives you the least amount of discomfort, whether it's bike riding, walking, swimming, or any of the other arthritis-friendly activities listed on page 44 in Chapter Three. The Arthritis Rx exercise program has been studied in a clinical trial with the proven effects of reducing pain and significantly decreasing reliance on pain medications. The Arthritis Rx Diet combined with the recommended daily exercise regimen in Part Three of this book can also contribute to weight loss.

## A YOUNG TENNIS PRO WITH A BAD HIP

A leading professional tennis player I'll call Jeff came to see me complaining of severe groin pain, which is the way hip arthritis usually presents itself. It's a bit unusual for someone in his late twenties to be suffering from arthritis, but Jeff had hip impingement syndrome—a bony protuberance in the hip bone that slowly wears away the cartilage. We have learned more about this condition in the last few years. The most common congenital problem is hip dysplasia, where the bone doesn't sit well in the socket. But the deleterious effects of Jeff's impingement had been exacerbated by his years of playing tennis on the professional circuit, and he had been experiencing a great deal of pain for the last couple of years. Even before the groin pain became noticeable, he had begun losing range of motion, which is also typical of this kind of arthritis.

By the time Jeff came to me, he had already tried a number of anti-inflammatory medications, but was having a serious problem with stomach pain from the NSAIDs, and the COX-2 inhibitors, which are supposed to be easier on the stomach but were no longer giving him much relief. I suggested that he follow the anti-inflammatory properties of my Arthritis Rx Diet, and he also began taking a combination of glucosamine, chondroitin sulfate, and ginger in the same proportions as Zingerflex. But what also struck me was that Jeff lacked core strength. The arthritis and loss of motion had contributed to an overall loss of muscle strength that can be devastating to any professional athlete. So along with modifying his diet to include more anti-inflammatory foods and supplements, I had him work on core strength by following the Arthritis Rx exercises. The combined program provided a synergistic result. The supplements and change of diet helped to reduce the pain of inflammation, allowing him to exercise harder. And because Jeff was such a well-conditioned athlete, he progressed to Series C in just a few weeks. I don't normally recommend such a rapid progression. Ideally, you should spend at least one month on each series, and most people don't even need to go beyond Series A to remain pain-free. But in Jeff's case I made an exception, and the results were startling. In two or three months his symptoms were reduced by 50 percent. His dependence on anti-inflammatories went from taking them five or seven days a week to just two days a week. And as his pain decreased and his range of motion improved, he was able to hit the ball much harder.

You might think that Jeff made such rapid progress only because he is a professional athlete and has the luxury of working with a coach and a personal trainer. But his strength-and-conditioning coach and the trainer didn't know what to treat because they weren't evaluating him from a medical viewpoint. Another reason Jeff's pain decreased is that his balance improved. The technical term for this kind of balance is proprioception, your ability to sense your joints in space. Stand on one leg and then close your eyes and you will immediately discover how hard it is to keep your balance. The nerve receptors in your foot, ankle, and leg are making hundreds of adjustments each second, triangulated by your eye's perception of spatial depth—your vertical body's relationship to the horizontal plane of the floor. That proprioceptive ability degenerates in an arthritic joint because inflammation inhibits the receptors. But exercise reactivates them, which is why it is so important to have a regular exercise regimen designed not only to strengthen your joints but also to reestablish your sense of balance and coordination.

Whether you need medication, integrative medicine, non-surgical procedures, or invasive surgery to correct an advanced stage of arthritis, it is important to continue with Stage One care during these other treatments. You should also resume the Arthritis Rx Plan after surgery to enhance recovery and prevent future problems. Some people may add heat and ice to the basic components of Stage One care, both of which reduce pain and stiffness in individual joints.

Now that you have a sense of the overall Arthritis Rx Plan, I'll go into each of the elements of the plan in much greater detail. I begin with the Arthritis Rx Diet, proceed to a discussion of the Arthritis Rx supplement Zingerflex, and then lead you through the Arthritis Rx Exercises with step-by-step instructions and accompanying photographs. By the time you are finished with Parts Two and Three of this book, you will have taken the most important steps to taking charge of your own arthritis care.

# CHAPTER FIVE

# THE ARTHRITIS Rx DIET

Hippocrates, the father of Western medicine, said, "Let your food be your medicine, and your medicine be your food." Nonetheless, too few physicians today follow this sage advice, or even seem aware of it. Nutritional counseling ought to be part of every discussion of healing chronic diseases such as arthritis because another old saying is also true: You are what you eat. Research has shown that the everyday decisions you make regarding the kind and amount of food you consume have a significant impact on your health. Food provides more than energy for your body to function. It also contains vital nutrients, including vitamins and minerals that are critical for the well-being of your bones, and substances that can slow down natural processes like inflammation that play key roles in the development of many diseases, including arthritis.

But if you are like many people with arthritis, you are probably skeptical about the impact of nutrition on the health of your joints. Even if you accept the concept, you may have lots of questions about what foods to eat. You may also wonder whether you will be able to eat tasty foods and still control your weight. But my research and clinical experience with hundreds of arthritis patients have shown that improving your nutrition will help you feel better and reduce your risk for complications, not only of arthritis but also of life-threatening illnesses such as heart disease, diabetes, and cancer.


## INFLAMMATION AND DISEASE

Nutrition is receiving more attention these days because research has found that it has a direct impact on inflammation, the body's natural response to irritation, injury, and infection. But in order to understand the connection, you first need to have a working knowledge of what inflammation is and how it functions in the human body. Simply put, inflammation is the self-protective process that occurs when you are injured. For instance, when you cut a finger, white blood cells rush to the site to kill the invading bacteria and wall off the area. The liquid component of the blood causes the tissue to swell and the injured skin to look puffy and red. This process has many positive effects: It slows bleeding and clears away debris from the destroyed tissue. If the tissues are irrevocably damaged, the inflammation process produces scar tissue that keeps foreign invaders out.

Unfortunately, you can have too much of a good thing, and inflammation also has a downside. Sometimes the process continues long after it is needed. In autoimmune disorders, the body's defense mechanisms wrongly destroy normal tissue, which often leads to other diseases. These overreactions of the autoimmune system may be the result of genetic predisposition, environmental toxins (contaminants in the air and water), or the food we eat. Chronic inflammation is dangerous because it harms tissues and makes them vulnerable to more serious ailments. Continued inflammation can attract white blood cells, LDL cholesterol, and blood platelets to artery walls, causing a buildup of plaque that often leads to heart disease and stroke.

As it turns out, heart disease researchers were among the first to discover that inflammation can play a destructive role in our health. Until the 1990s, physicians assumed that heart disease was a "plumbing problem": Cholesterol gradually builds up and clogs the arteries with plaque so that they can no longer deliver oxygen-rich blood to the heart and brain. Eventually, the plaque bursts, cutting off the blood supply and resulting in a heart attack or stroke. This theory, however, didn't explain why many people who had normal cholesterol and blood pressure, and a low risk of cardiovascular disease, died of heart attacks and strokes. Recent studies have identified a new culprit, called C-reactive protein (CRP), a naturally occurring chemical in the blood that is involved in fighting infection. Scientists believe that high levels of CRP in the blood can cause small amounts of plaque in the arteries to break away, becoming a clot that leads to heart attacks and strokes. CRP is also seen as both a promoter of inflammation and a major cause of heart disease, a fact that underlies the current perception that heart disease is essentially an inflammatory process.

One of the most important studies was done by researchers at Harvard Medical School, who followed the development of heart disease among 28,000 women over an eight-year period. They found that those with the highest levels of CRP were twice as likely to die from heart attacks and strokes as those with normal CRP levels. Even more amazing was the finding that half of heart attacks and strokes occurred in those with seemingly safe levels of cholesterol. Smaller studies in men showed similar results. Elevated levels of CRP have been found in cases of arthritis, cancer, and Alzheimer's disease.

Inflammation may also be implicated in the development of diabetes and may be another risk factor for cardiovascular disease, kidney failure, and nerve damage. Diabetes is a disease in which too much sugar accumulates in the bloodstream, rather than being carried to cells throughout the body. Some studies suggest that elevated CRP levels reduce the body's ability to produce insulin, the hormone that it needs to transform the glucose in food into energy. (Insulin is secreted by the pancreas in sufficient levels to maintain the proper balance of blood sugar throughout the day, and is essential for the metabolism of protein and fat. Insufficient production of insulin can lead to the onset of type 2 diabetes.)

The theory that inflammation and cancer are linked has been circulated since the 1860s, when the German pathologist Rudolph Virchow speculated that cancerous tumors begin at the sites of wounds that never heal. Geneticists in the twentieth century theorized that genetic mutations and inflammation work together to transform normal cells into deadly cancers. Other researchers are investigating the possibility that inflammation may be implicated in other diseases, such as asthma and Alzheimer's disease.

Even stronger evidence for the role of inflammation in promoting disease comes from years of studying arthritis, especially rheumatoid arthritis (RA). The exact cause of RA is unknown, and according to the Arthritis Foundation, researchers are now debating whether RA is one disease or several different diseases with common features. What they agree on is that the body's immune system plays an important role, and so RA is referred to as an autoimmune disease. People with RA have an abnormal immune system response that leads their systems to mistake the body's healthy tissue for a foreign invader and attack it, including the tissue lining the joints. Once the response is under way, fluid builds up in the tissues, causing swelling. As the tissues swell, the pressure builds, leading to pain and stiffness. The inflamed tissues also release enzymes that may destroy bone and cartilage, resulting in further damage and a vicious cycle that can lead to more pain.

Recent studies, however, have found that there is a window of opportunity in early RA when this destructive inflammation process can be halted. Administering powerful drugs, such as Enbrel and Remicaid, during the first few months after a diagnosis protects the joints so that pain and stiffness are avoided. That same inflammatory process also seems to be responsible for a greater risk of cardiovascular disease in people with rheumatoid arthritis. Women with RA had twice the risk of heart attack as women without the condition, according to the Nurses' Health Study, a twenty-year investigation of over 114,000 women followed by researchers at the Harvard Medical School. Women who had had rheumatoid arthritis for more than ten years had the highest risk.

Of course, people afflicted with osteoarthritis also suffer from the pain of inflammation, and so it's important for them to follow a regimen that will help reduce inflammation as much as possible. One of the most effective pathways to pain reduction is through modifying what we eat.

# INFLAMMATION AND DIET

Perhaps the most radical medical insight to come out of all the research into inflammation is the role that certain foods can play in initiating the process. Researchers now believe that certain foods labeled "pro-inflammatory" cause the body's natural defense system to respond in much the same way it would to a wound or other injury. They theorize that, for a variety of reasons, cells produce free oxygen radicals—negatively charged oxygen atoms or molecules that are created when oxygen interacts with certain kinds of molecules. Free radicals lack an electron in their outer shell and seek to bond with other atoms or molecules to stabilize themselves. Once formed, these highly reactive radicals can start a chain reaction, like dominoes, forcing other molecules to become unstable in turn. They build up over time and promote inflammation, cause cartilage to lose its ability to bounce back, artery walls to lose their ability to resist plaque, and airways to lose their tendency to remain open. Some free radicals arise normally during metabolism or are created by the body's immune system cells to neutralize viruses and bacteria. The body can usually process free radicals with the help of its own supply of antioxidants, substances that act as scavengers and bind to free radicals, which bond with the atoms and render them harmless. Certain foods also contain antioxidants, helping to prevent cell and tissue damage that could lead to cellular degeneration and disease. But if enough antioxidants are not available, or if free radical production becomes excessive because of environmental factors such as pollution, radiation, cigarette smoke, herbicides, or pro-inflammatory foods, serious damage can occur. Free radicals also attack cell membranes and red blood cells, and cause damage in DNA/RNA strands, triggering mutations in tissue, blood vessels, and skin.

Extensive studies show that free radicals not only develop in the body due to exposure to toxic chemicals in air, food, and water, but are also formed by the body's normal chemical processes, including metabolism of polyunsaturated fats. Polyunsaturated fats—the kind present in most vegetable oils and margarine—have been repeatedly tied to risk of cancer and heart disease. New evidence links exposure to free radicals with premature aging and autoimmune diseases such as rheumatoid arthritis, as well as Parkinson's, Lou Gehrig's, and Alzheimer's diseases.

While some fats produce inflammation, others, mainly the essential fatty acids (EFAs), inhibit it. These fatty acids are called essential because our body cannot produce them, so we must get them from food or supplements. The omega-3 fatty acids found in foods including cold-water fish (such as salmon, mackerel, sardines, herring, bass, swordfish, and tuna) and in flaxseed, walnuts, and dark green leafy vegetables (including kale, spinach, chard, broccoli, and dark green lettuces) have been shown to discourage the production of inflammatory chemicals that harm the joints and other parts of the body. These EFAs appear to turn off inflammatory re-actions when the body no longer needs them, and so keep the inflammation process from running amok. They also contribute to the creation of a variety of powerful anti-inflammatory substances. The fat from which all the omega-3s derive is alpha-linolenic acid, which can be found in flaxseed oil and dark green leafy vegetables. (Another family of EFAs called omega-9s work with the omega-3 acids to inhibit in-flammation. They are found most prominently in olive oil, avocados, and macadamia nuts.)

By contrast, saturated omega-6 fatty acids, found in red meat and other animal products and in many vegetable oils used in cooking and baking, promote inflam-mation. Although linoleic acid, the basis of all the other omega-6 fatty acids, is es-sential for health, it represents another instance of having too much of a good thing. Our diet is overloaded with omega-6 foods, including the omnipresent vegetable oils (corn, sunflower, safflower, peanut) that are used to fry foods and make potato and corn chips and are added to most processed foods, commercial salad dressings, microwavable food, frozen food, and many brand-name breakfast bars and candy bars. Until about one hundred years ago, our ancestors lived well on a diet in which omega-6 and omega-3 fatty acids were in balance. The ideal ratio of omega-6 to omega-3 fats is between 1:1 and 2:1, which has been our traditional diet for many thousands of years. Today the ratio averages more than 20:1, which is dangerous to health. A study in the January 2002 *American Journal of Clinical Nutrition* determined that the omega-6 fats in these oils increased inflammation in heart cells. One of the by-products of linoleic acid in the body is arachidonic acid, which contributes to the formation of eicosanoids, compounds that cause inflammation, such as prostaglandin $E_2$. So, eating more of the good omega-3 fats and less of the bad omega-6 fats is believed to slow the development and progression of inflammation.

There are other sound reasons for not eating snack chips. Acrylamide, an industrial chemical used in plastics, pesticides, and sewage treatment, can also occur when certain carbohydrate-rich foods are fried, baked, or roasted at high temperatures. These foods include most potato and corn chips, pretzels, crackers, and fast food French fries. Acrylamide can cause cancer in laboratory animals at high doses, although it is not clear whether it causes cancer at the much lower levels in food. Nonetheless, the UN Food and Agriculture Organization and the World Health Organization warn that acrylamide may be a public health concern, and have called for continued efforts to reduce acrylamide in food. Canola oil, a form of cooking and salad oil derived from rapeseed (a plant also cultivated for the production of animal feed and biodiesel fuel), has been the subject of a great deal of controversy and conflicting claims. It has very little omega-6 fatty acid compared with corn, safflower, and peanut oils, but like them it is often used in hydrogenated form in processed foods. Canola oil (the name derives from Canada, where most of the rapeseed used to make it was grown) is produced by artificial industrial processing, and even though it is low in omega-6 acids, I'm not comfortable recommending its use.

| Omega-3 and Omega-9 Foods (Highly Recommended) | Omega-6 Foods (Avoid) |
| --- | --- |
| Fatty cold-water fish | Red meat |
| Flaxseed oil, olive oil | Corn, safflower, sunflower, soy, and peanut oils |
| Avocados, walnuts, macadamia nuts | |
| Broccoli, kale, collards, spinach, chard | Fast food |
| Cabbage, cauliflower, kohlrabi | Commercial baked goods |
| | Deep-fried foods |

Many vitamins and minerals have been found to protect the body against inflammation. These include vitamins A, C, D, and E, folate (a B vitamin), and the mineral selenium. Vitamin C is the most abundant water-soluble antioxidant in the body. Present in citrus fruits and juices, green peppers, cabbage, spinach, broccoli, kale, cantaloupe, kiwi, and strawberries, it repairs and builds collagen, the primary component of cartilage. Vitamin D (found in whole grains, dark green leafy vegetables, nuts and seeds, herring, eggs, milk, organ meats, and sweet potatoes) appears to help bones retain calcium so that they can absorb shock. A 1999 study published in *Arthritis & Rheumatism* showed evidence that this vitamin protects against hip arthritis. Vitamin E, the most abundant fat-soluble antioxidant in the body (present in nuts, seeds, fish oils, whole grains, and apricots), helps shut off genes involved in inflammation and significantly reduces CRP levels. One of the most efficient chain-breaking antioxidants available, vitamin E defends against lipid peroxidation, the creation of unstable molecules containing more oxygen than is usual.

These vitamins are also abundant in a wide variety of whole foods, as we will see in the discussion of highly recommended foods. What whole foods have that many vitamin supplements lack, moreover, is a wealth of vitaminlike antioxidant nutrients such as flavonoids and carotenoids, compounds that lend color to fruits and vegetables. A flavonoid such as quercetin, found in onions and apples, helps inhibit inflammation. The carotenoids include beta-carotene, a powerful inflammation fighter found in carrots, apricots, squash, and other yellow-orange fruits and vegetables, as well as liver, egg yolk, milk, butter, spinach, broccoli, and yams. Whole foods contain complexes of these nutrients that appear to work more successfully in concert with one another than separately in extracted supplements. That said, it's important to eat as wide an array of healthful foods as possible. Following is a list of the anti- and pro-inflammatory foods to keep in mind as you read on.

| Anti-inflammatory Foods (Recommended) | Pro-inflammatory Foods (Not Recommended) |
|---|---|
| Cold-water fish (salmon, tuna, mackerel, sardines, bass, anchovies) | Red meat, hot dogs, hamburgers, fast food, frozen dinners |
| Fruits (apples, oranges, berries, avocados) | Chips, packaged snack foods |
| Whole grains (wheat, brown rice, oats, quinoa) | Refined grain products (white bread, pasta) |
| Dark-green leafy vegetables (broccoli, kale, chard, spinach, lettuce) | Most commercial, non-organic salad dressings and energy/breakfast bars (see pp. 69–72) |
| Olive oil, flaxseed oil, borage oil, evening primrose oil | Vegetable oils (corn, sunflower, safflower, peanut, coconut, palm) |
| Soy products (soymilk, soy cheese) | Dairy products (unless low-fat) |
| Walnuts, butternuts, soy nuts, flaxseed | Dry-roasted peanuts, beer nuts |
| Green tea, oolong tea, water, mineral water | Carbonated drinks, juice drinks, soda |
| Spices (ginger, turmeric) | Refined sugars, sweets (candy, cookies, cake chocolate) |

## THE ANTI-INFLAMMATORY DIET

Your approach to eating should be a little like having a diversified stock portfolio that doesn't rely too heavily on any one market sector. The best dietary advice seems to be to eat a balanced diet that includes specific anti-inflammatory foods, in conjunction with maintaining a healthy weight with the help of portion control and regular exercise. I advise my patients to follow the anti-inflammatory diet, a variation of the Unified Dietary Guidelines that any healthy adult should follow to maintain health and prevent disease. In March 2005, the National Institutes of Health, the American Heart Association, the American Cancer Society, and the American Academy of Pediatrics created the guidelines to decrease the risk of life-threatening heart attacks, strokes, cancer, and other conditions. They recommend these daily limits for adults, based on a 2,000-calorie diet:

**1. Total fat should make up 20 to 35 percent of calories (44 to 78 grams).** The typical American diet gets 40 to 59 percent of calories from fat. Moreover, many of those fat calories come not from the natural fats in many foods that are beneficial to health (fat is a major source of energy for the body and aids in the absorption of vitamins A, D, E, and K, and carotenoids), but from the hydrogenated fats in most processed and fast foods.

**2. Saturated fat should be less than 10 percent of total calories (fewer than 22 grams).** Saturated fats are those that are either solid or almost solid at room temperature. You can readily see them when fats congeal in the pan or on top of soups or stews made with meat or poultry. Dairy products also contain saturated fats, as do most processed and fast foods. Saturated fats tend to raise cholesterol levels and therefore increase the risk of heart disease.

**3. Trans fats should be as low as possible, less than 1 percent of total calories (fewer than 2 grams).** Fats and oils that contain mostly unsaturated fat can be made more saturated through a process called "hydrogenation," whereby they are infused with hydrogen to make them more stable and increase their shelf life. This process that turns liquid oil into stick margarine or shortening and prevents the oil in foods like peanut butter from separating creates what are known as trans fats. Although these hydrogenated or partially hydrogenated oils allow food manufacturers to produce larger quantities at one time and grocery stores to keep them on the shelf longer without spoilage, they are almost invariably bad for your health and can cause weight gain. Since 1993, the Food and Drug Administration has required amounts of saturated fat and dietary cholesterol to be listed on food labels. As of January 1, 2006, the FDA required listing of trans fat as well. When you see "hydrogenated" or "partially hydrogenated" oil of any kind among the ingredients on a food product label, you're better off leaving it on the shelf. It will enjoy a longer life by itself, and so will you.

**4. Cholesterol should be fewer than 300 milligrams.** Many nutritionists distinguish between LDL (low-density lipoprotein) cholesterol and HDL (high-density lipoprotein) cholesterol. The former is often referred to as bad cholesterol, although it actually serves a useful function in the body, carrying fat-soluble nutrients such as vitamin E in the blood. But according to the American Heart Association, too much LDL cholesterol in the blood can slowly build up in the inner walls of the arteries that feed the heart and brain. Together with other substances, it can form a thick, hard deposit called plaque that can clog those arteries, a condition known as artherosclerosis. If a clot forms and blocks a narrowed artery, it can cause a heart attack or stroke. HDL cholesterol is known as good cholesterol because a high level of it seems to protect against heart attack. Medical experts think that HDL may carry cholesterol away from the arteries and back to the liver, where it passes out of the body, and that it removes excess cholesterol from arterial plaque, slowing the buildup.

## WHAT SHOULD I EAT?

The anti-inflammatory diet follows these guidelines and is designed to reduce the factors that cause inflammation and high levels of LDL cholesterol by emphasizing plant foods: primarily fruits, vegetables, and whole grains. You don't have to be suffering from arthritis to want to gravitate to the foods that help fight inflammation and reduce the pain associated with it. Indeed, if you are reading this book because a member of your family has arthritis and you want to help, you can be confident that if you follow these nutritional guidelines to encourage your family member to do likewise, you will be improving the length and quality of your own life as well. For example, eating five or more servings of fruits and vegetables each day will help reduce inflammation and the pain of arthritis. But a study published in the June 2004 issue of *Archives of Ophthalmology* shows that eating three or more servings of fruit a day may also lower the risk of age-related macular degeneration, the primary cause of vision loss in older adults, by 36 percent compared to people who consume only one serving of fruit daily. Although I have emphasized those foods that especially fight inflammation and the resultant symptoms of arthritis, many of the same foods have been proven to help prevent heart disease, stroke, diabetes, cancer, Alzheimer's disease, and a host of gastrointestinal ailments from ulcers to constipation.

As I stated earlier, to get the most out of the protective, antioxidant qualities of these foods, you should eat a varied diet. Most people like to have different main courses throughout the week but end up eating the same few fruits and vegetables (if they eat any at all). Certain foods are less expensive and taste better when they are in season and locally grown. Organic produce is more likely to have been cultivated in soil that isn't depleted of essential nutrients than the crops grown by large agribusiness farms, and so may contain higher levels of these nutrients and not be tainted by pesticides. Organic fruits and vegetables also tend to cost more and may be harder to find, although many supermarkets now carry at least a small selection of organic products, including grains and prepared foods, and these are worth seeking out. Unlike the non-organic salad dressings, breakfast bars, frozen foods, fruit drinks, and other prepared items in most grocery stores, the ones you'll find in health food stores are usually free of partially hydrogenated oils, omega-6 oils, refined sugars, and chemical additives that promote inflammation and are generally toxic to your health. But it's still important to check the label! (For example, frozen fruits and vegetables can be a convenient way to keep supplies on hand, but many commercial brands add unnecessary sugar, corn oil, or preservatives, so read the ingredients carefully.)

## ALWAYS READ THE LABEL!

Discovering what is actually in the food you buy in stores is often complicated by the fact that some labels are designed to be misleading or to emphasize apparently desirable facts while failing to mention less appealing information. Cookies and baked goods labeled "cholesterol free" or "fat free" often have a high caloric content, and consuming these products with abandon can lead to unexpected weight gain. Some products that trumpet "all-natural ingredients" may be loaded with fats and sugars that are natural but nonetheless unhealthful. What's a poor consumer to do?

To begin with, distinguish between the **nutrition facts** and the **list of ingredients**. The **Nutrition Facts Panel**, or NFP, created by the U.S. Food and Drug Administration (FDA), lists calories and fat calories (if any); the amount of protein, fats (now including trans fat), cholesterol, carbohydrates, dietary fiber, sugars, sodium, and certain other key nutritional components in grams; and the percent of Daily Value (formerly the Recommended Daily Allowance) that these components offer in a single serving. This may be helpful information, but it can be complicated to read—the FDA has a lengthy Web page that explains in detail how to interpret it. The best way to use the NFP is to multiply the number of servings listed at the top of the label by the number of calories listed below it. For instance, a 13-ounce bag of a popular corn chip lists the following information:

Serving size 1 oz.
Number of servings 13
Calories (per serving) 140
Calories from fat 60

Simple math tells you that thirteen servings multiplied by 140 calories means that this average-sized bag of chips contains 1,820 calories—almost your entire recommended daily value of 2,000 calories. Further, 780 of those calories are from fat, or roughly 43 percent—well over the 20 to 35 percent recommended by the Unified Dietary Guidelines.

The **list of ingredients**, usually found near the nutrition facts at the bottom of the label, is much more straightforward and easier to comprehend. By law it must list all ingredients in order of predominance, with the ingredients used in the greatest amount first, followed in descending order by those in smaller amounts. Thus a bottle of lemonade might list water first, followed by sugar, lemon juice concentrate, citric acid, natural and/or artificial flavors, and perhaps preservatives. The ingredients on that bag of corn chips above include vegetable oils (soybean and safflower), salt, partially hydrogenated soybean oil, MSG (monosodium glutamate), sugar, and dextrose—a simple sugar more commonly known as glucose, which can lead to a spike in blood sugar levels. You don't need any of those ingredients.

Reading the ingredients of most juice drinks will quickly tell you that they are made up mostly of water and sugar, with little real fruit juice, which is one good reason to avoid them at all costs. Many commercial cereal manufacturers have jumped on the whole-grain bandwagon, and that's a good development. But if the ingredient listed after whole-grain oats is sugar, as it often is, you won't be doing yourself or your kids any favors by purchasing that product. And if you find hydrogenated or partially hydrogenated oils anywhere on the list of ingredients, choose a different product.

Breakfast bars and so-called energy bars represent an especially challenging temptation. These products promise to deliver enough protein and carbs to get you going in the morning or pick you up in the middle of your workday with just a few quick bites. And yet the first ingredient listed on one very popular energy bar is high-fructose corn syrup! That provides a big burst of calories and pro-inflammatory omega-6 without much nutrition to show for it. The same goes for a leading brand-name breakfast drink that lists sugar as its first ingredient. As we have known for some time, those quick sugar highs are often followed by an energy letdown.

If you are looking for reliable, slow-burning energy, you'll do better with bars that contain only whole grains, dried fruits, nuts, or seeds, and maybe a natural sweetener such as unrefined cane juice, honey, or agave nectar. The carbs in these kinds of energy bars burn more slowly and provide energy without creating a big spike in blood-sugar levels. Most energy bars available in health food stores (many of which can also be bought over the Internet) contain no hydrogenated oils, added sugar, corn syrup, corn oil, sulfured fruits, preservatives, or other undesirable ingredients. These bars are not a substitute for fresh fruits and vegetables, but they do represent a wholesome way to keep your energy level stable and satisfy hunger without harming your body. If the list of ingredients contains only organic flaxseed, organic apples, dates, sesame seeds, raisins, and agave nectar, the bar is probably all right.

Much the same is true for granola. This apparent product of the 1960s hippie subculture actually has roots going back to the founders of the Kellogg and Post cereal companies in the nineteenth century, who created similar cereals made of ground and baked whole grains that were quite healthful. Today so many versions are in the marketplace under the generic name "granola" that you have to read the labels carefully to make sure they really have whole grains and no added sugar or other adulterations. So beware of granolas marketed by the mainstream cereal companies, which are mainly designed to satisfy America's sweet tooth.

As a rule, if you are not buying packaged food products from reputable health food companies, you are probably ingesting unnecessary toxins with your food. Most commercial brands of boxed or canned chicken stock, for example, contain hydrolyzed soy protein and/or monosodium glutamate (MSG). The hydrolysis process used to produce hydrolyzed soy protein involves boiling soybeans in a vat of acid and then neutralizing the solution with a caustic soda. The resultant sludge is scraped off the top and dried. MSG is a neurotoxin that is known to cause headaches and other allergic reactions in many people. You'll also find sugar, corn oil, and MSG in many frozen foods, including fish sticks. Most commercial salad dressings contain hydrogenated vegetable oils, added sugar, and preservatives. You're much better off trying some of the many brands sold in health food stores and supermarket health sections, or making your own simple balsamic vinaigrette dressing. (See p. 116 for recipe.) But even some dressings sold in health food stores contain corn oil, so once again . . . always read the label.

## THE CARBOHYDRATE DILEMMA

Conflicting claims about the value of carbohydrates (carbs) versus protein and fats have succeeded in confusing many people about what they ought to eat. Even the USDA food pyramid has been criticized by reputable nutritionists for placing too much emphasis on grains, including breads, cereals, rice, and pasta, which are all high in carbs. Carbs in and of themselves aren't bad. Fruits, vegetables, and whole grains all have substantial amounts of carbs, which are a major source of energy for the body and brain. High-protein diets that discourage eating all carbs can leave people with low levels of energy. The problem with carbs comes from the over-refining of grains, a process that began early in the last century and that removes the essential nutritional elements (germ and bran). The kinds of carbs you want are the ones that are considered complex, meaning that it takes the body much longer to break them down into their essential sugars. The carbs in whole grains, for example, are nutritious because they provide slowly released fuel that staves off hunger while supplying the brain and body with plenty of energy, as well as valuable dietary fiber. These kinds of carbs are also called low-glycemic because the gradual release of sugars does not cause a dangerous spike in blood sugar levels. This puts less of a burden on the insulin-producing cells in the pancreas and keeps your energy level more stable.

The carbohydrates in many of the foods that abound today, such as bagels, doughnuts, muffins, pastries, cakes, and cookies, are much simpler in structure because of their refined ingredients. These high-glycemic carbs are converted to glucose very quickly and release large amounts of sugar into the bloodstream, providing an energy rush that is often followed by a plunge in energy levels and a craving for yet more carbs. One good way to regulate blood glucose is through exercise, which builds up muscles and makes them more energy-demanding. This in turn helps burn excess body fat and establishes a healthy body-fat percentage, as shown by the body mass index indicator described in Chapter Two. Another way to stabilize blood sugar levels is to eat primarily the kinds of low-glycemic complex carbohydrates contained in whole grains and many of the foods in the lists at the end of this chapter.

## DIETARY FIBER

In recent years, accumulating research has begun to suggest that sufficient dietary fiber may prevent cancer, diabetes, heart disease, and obesity. Because overweight and obese individuals tend to suffer much more from arthritis than others, it is crucially important that you get enough of the proper dietary fiber on a regular basis to help keep your weight down. Fiber used to be called roughage—bran muffins, fruits, and vegetables—and was believed to aid in digestion and in regulating bowel movements. But scientists and nutritionists have discovered that there is much more to fiber than just regularity. Fiber is an undigestible complex carbohydrate found in plants, rather than any single food or substance. Because your body can't absorb it, fiber has no caloric content. It also tends to fill the stomach and give you a feeling of fullness, so eating plenty of fiber is a great natural way to control your appetite.

There are two basic categories of fiber. **Water-soluble fibers**, found in certain fruits (apples, oranges, peaches, prunes, and grapes), oat bran, and beans, help lower blood cholesterol levels and normalize blood sugar levels, reducing the need for insulin production. **Insoluble fibers** (cellulose, hemicellulose, and lignin) do not dissolve in water; they help promote regularity by adding bulk to waste matter and moving it through the colon more quickly. This helps prevent constipation and may prevent colon cancer. You get insoluble fiber from fruits, vegetables, dried beans, seeds, popcorn, brown rice, and whole-grain products. (Many whole foods contain both kinds of fiber.) Although fiber is not considered an essential nutrient, the Surgeon General and professional health organizations recommend a daily diet containing 20 to 35 grams of fiber. On average, Americans consume about half this amount. You can build your daily fiber intake by eating more complex carbohydrates—fruits, vegetables, and whole grains—as opposed to refined sugar and flour, processed foods, and sodas. But increase your intake gradually over several weeks or you may experience diarrhea, gas, and bloating. As you eat more fiber, be sure to drink more water to help avoid stomach discomfort. Once you get your intake to the desired level, you should experience no discomfort at all. You can use fiber supplements if necessary, but it's better to get dietary fiber from whole foods that are also rich in vitamins, minerals, and phytonutrients.

## WHOLE FOODS TO FIGHT INFLAMMATION

The preponderance of research shows that the most vital foods contain an astonishing array of vitamins, minerals, nutrients, phytochemicals, and compounds such as flavonoids and carotenoids that are invaluable for health but difficult to get in supplement form. Supplements can help fill in some of the gaps, but there is just no adequate substitute for eating whole foods themselves. The most important foods for fighting inflammation and arthritis are fruits, vegetables, and cold-water fish.

### FRUITS AND VEGETABLES

Fruits and vegetables that have the richest colors, such as blueberries, strawberries, dark green kale, and spinach, are the highest in carotenoids and bioflavonoids, the powerful antioxidants that help prevent oxidation and inflammation. Bioflavonoids, which are responsible for the colors in fruits and vegetables, have inherent anti-inflammatory properties. Flavonoids are gaining increased recognition as part of a healthy anti-inflammatory diet that, along with supplements, will play a key role in

# SERVING SIZE

A serving of any food is probably much smaller than you think. For one thing, the Food and Drug Administration (FDA) and United States Department of Agriculture (USDA) use different protocols for determining serving size. The USDA is responsible for creating and revising the food pyramid, now called MyPyramid, whereas the FDA is responsible for the listing of a product's nutritional information on the Nutrition Facts Panel (NFP) found on food packaging. The important thing to know is that the USDA-recommended serving size of fruits is one medium-sized piece—an apple, banana, kiwi, or pear; ½ cup chopped or loose fruit (such as blueberries); or ¾ cup of pure fruit juice. For vegetables, a serving means one cup of leafy greens like kale or lettuce; ½ cup of denser veggies, such as peas or squash; or ¾ cup of vegetable juice. For grains, the standard is 1 ounce (one slice) of bread or cold cereal, such as granola, or ½ cup cooked cereal, rice, or pasta. When it comes to fish, poultry, or meat, a serving consists of 3 ounces, or about half the usual portion. Given the serving size for fruits and vegetables, five servings a day are not that difficult to consume.

You should allocate two-thirds of your plate to plant-based foods. The other third should contain fish, lean meat, or skinless poultry—all rich in protein that is needed to build and maintain tissues. Tofu, beans, dried peas, or lentils can be used as alternatives to animal fats; they have sufficient protein but are low in saturated fat. Red meat contains high levels of arachidonic acid, which increases inflammation, so removing meat from the diet decreases the levels of pro-inflammatory compounds in the body. Caffeine, fried foods, carbonated drinks, and alcohol greatly increase oxidation and free radicals, both of which initiate the inflammatory process.

managing arthritis in the future. It pays to eat foods of different colors occasionally as pigmentation can indicate the presence of different nutrients. One orange-red carotenoid (beta-cryptoxanthin) found in the highest amounts in like-colored foods, such as pumpkin, papaya, red bell peppers, tangerines, and peaches, may significantly lower the risk of developing lung cancer.

I recommend that my patients eat five servings of fruits and vegetables a day. These servings will help them not only manage their arthritis but also reduce their risk of diabetes, heart disease, certain cancers, and obesity. Fat cells in the body produce proteins called cytokines, which encourage inflammation, perhaps providing a link between obesity, chronic inflammation, and type 2 diabetes. Because obesity also puts more stress on the weight-bearing joints, it exacerbates arthritis pain.

## NIGHTSHADE PLANTS

Of course, there is no guarantee that either consuming or giving up any one food or group of foods will help all or most people with arthritis. You have to try various things and discover what makes you feel best. Some people feel stronger when they give up animal protein and eat a vegetarian diet, while others feel weak and undernourished. Some feel better when they eliminate gluten, found in wheat, rye, barley, and oats. For others, the answer is giving up all dairy products or fermented foods such as soy sauce, beer, and wine. And for a certain number of people with arthritis, perhaps as high as 20 percent by some estimates, foods in the nightshade family exacerbate their condition.

The nightshades (*Solanaceae*) include tomatoes, white potatoes, eggplant, and peppers (bell, cayenne, chili, paprika, and pimiento but not black pepper), as well as tobacco and belladonna. Through the fifteenth century, most Europeans considered these foods toxic. Yet when Columbus discovered America, he found the inhabitants living healthy lives consuming all of these substances. They soon became important food crops, especially the potato, whose high levels of vitamin C and niacin cannot be destroyed by boiling. But all nightshades contain a chemical alkaloid called solanine that, if not destroyed in the intestines, could be toxic for some people. A horticulturist named Dr. Norman Childers hypothesized that some individuals whose intestinal tracts are unable to destroy solanine may become arthritic as a result. According to the *Journal of Neurological and Orthopedic Medical Surgery* (1993), total avoidance of nightshades, with other minor dietary adjustments, has resulted in positive to marked improvement in arthritis. But the nightshade-avoidance diet has not yet had a strict clinical test. Once again, the key is to use common sense. If you eat a lot of tomatoes, potatoes, peppers, and eggplant and you have arthritis pain, try removing them completely from your diet for six months and see what results. (Six months is the recommended span for most elimination diets.) But keep in mind that many prepared sauces, salad dressings, salsas, and relishes may contain versions of these foods, so read labels carefully. Because all these foods contain valuable nutrients, don't stop eating them if you don't have to.

## FATTY COLD-WATER FISH

Omega-3 fatty acids are found in cold-water fish such as salmon, herring, tuna, anchovies, bluefish, and sardines, as well as in flaxseed, walnuts, and dark green vegetables including collards, kale, chard, and spinach. But cold-water fish are the only abundant source of the two most effective omega-3 unsaturated fatty acids known as eicosapentaenoic acid, or EPA, and docosahexaenoic acid, or DHA. These acids have been shown to reduce the risk of blood clotting, abnormal heart rhythms, and the creation of arterial plaque, and to be extremely effective in fighting inflammation. A study carried out at the University of Pittsburgh School of Medicine in 2004 placed one hundred twenty patients on fish oil supplements containing the omega-3 essential fatty acids for treatment of their neck and low-back pain, which resulted from disk disease and arthritis. Of those patients, 59 percent experienced decreased joint pain and 68 percent were able to discontinue taking NSAIDs. The study also found that most patients had no side effects and that 86 percent planned to continue the use of fish oil supplements. An earlier study in 1994 in Denmark found that patients with rheumatoid arthritis who ate 4 ounces of these fish every day for six months reported less stiffness and pain, and fewer swollen joints than rheumatoid arthritis patients who didn't eat fish. (Another benefit for women may be reduced risk of breast cancer. In animal studies, a high intake of omega-3 fatty acids from fish oils has been shown to slow the development and growth of breast tumors.)

Some shellfish are also helpful in fighting inflammation. Scallops are a good source of vitamin $B_{12}$, which helps convert homocysteine into benign chemicals. High levels of homocysteine are associated with an increased risk of atherosclerosis, heart attack, and stroke, as well as osteoporosis. Scallops also have good amounts of omega-3 fatty acids and magnesium, which help lower blood pressure (by relaxing blood vessels). Dieters have known for some time that shrimp are low in both calories and fat and yet are a good source of protein (as well as vitamins D and $B_{12}$). And at least one study has shown that eating a diet in which a serving of shrimp was substituted for eggs lowered levels of triglycerides, the chemical form in which fat is contained and conveyed in the body. So both of these forms of protein offer an alternative to red meat as well as a change from fish.

In addition, to be sure that you get enough essential omega-3 fatty acids in your diet, you can take fish oil supplements that contain EPA and DHA. A typical softgel supplement with 1,000 mg of fish oil might contain 180 mg of EPA and 120 mg of DHA. I recommend taking 2 or 3 grams a day, especially on days when you don't eat any fish.

## SHOULD I BE CONCERNED
## ABOUT MERCURY IN FISH?

Since I am advising readers to eat a good amount of fish every week, I should address the concerns that many people have about the levels of mercury in fish. Mercury occurs naturally in the environment and is also released into the air through industrial pollution. It then falls from the air and accumulates in rivers, streams, lakes, and oceans, where it combines with bacteria to produce methylmercury. This kind of mercury is harmful to an unborn baby or young child. Fish absorb the methylmercury as they feed in these waters and it builds up in them. It accumulates more in larger, predatory fish, such as swordfish and sharks, because they live longer and have more time to absorb methylmercury. The latest guidelines from the FDA (and EPA) published in March 2004 are for the most part favorable about eating fish, with a few caveats, which are worth quoting in detail:

> For most people, the risk from mercury by eating fish and shellfish is not a health concern. Yet, some fish and shellfish contain higher levels of mercury that may harm an unborn baby or young child's developing nervous system. The risks from mercury in fish and shellfish depend on the amount of fish and shellfish eaten and the levels of mercury in the fish and shellfish. Therefore, the Food and Drug Administration (FDA) and the Environmental Protection Agency (EPA) are advising women who may become pregnant, pregnant women, nursing mothers, and young children to avoid some types of fish and eat fish and shellfish that are lower in mercury.
>
> ["What You Need to Know About Mercury in Fish and Shellfish,"
> EPA-823-R-04-005, March 2004,
> http://www.cfsan.fda.gov/~dms/admehg3.html]

The advisory warns women and young children as defined above against eating shark, swordfish, king mackerel, or tilefish because they contain high levels of mercury. It suggests eating up to 12 ounces a week of a variety of fish and shellfish that are lower in mercury, including shrimp, canned light tuna, salmon, pollock, and catfish. Albacore ("white") tuna has more mercury than canned light tuna, and so should be limited to no more than 6 ounces a week.

# DAIRY AND EGGS

Nutritionists differ in their opinion of the healthfulness of dairy products. We have been warned not only that dairy tends to increase cholesterol levels in the blood but also that the lactose in milk products, a form of sugar, can promote weight gain. But we should also be aware of the benefits of some forms of dairy, as well as eggs. A number of recent studies have shown that eggs do not substantially affect levels of cholesterol in most people and that they may actually reduce the risk of heart attack and stroke because proteins present in egg yolk help to prevent blood clots. More important, eggs are a good source of both vitamin $B_{12}$ and choline, an essential nutrient required by the body to make several important compounds necessary for healthy cell membranes. A single egg also provides 11 percent of the daily requirement of protein—necessary to create the amino acids we need to survive—yet contains only 68 calories. If you buy organic eggs produced by free-range chickens, you will avoid the negative effects of the hormones that are also present in most commercially produced beef and pork. Some dairy farmers now feed their hens grains rich in omega-3 to add another source of this valuable element to our diet.

Some forms of dairy, including milk, yogurt, and cheese, have some benefit as well when consumed in moderation. For example, a study published in the *New England Journal of Medicine* in 2004 points out that eating more dairy foods decreases the risk of gout, a common form of arthritis whose onset typically involves the big toe. Cheese and yogurt also induce feelings of satiation that help control the appetite and the desire to eat snacks loaded with omega-6, such as corn chips and potato chips. Dairy products can be highly caloric, however, so try to use fat-free or low-fat varieties of milk, cheese, and yogurt to help prevent weight gain.

## WHAT IS AN OMEGA-3 EGG?

A growing number of egg producers feed their hens special diets to produce eggs with enhanced amounts of omega-3 fatty acids. These eggs contain 100 to 200 mg of omega-3s (three to six times that of a normal egg), which helps to ameliorate one of the negative aspects of commercially produced eggs: the undesirable omega-6 to omega-3 ratio of many egg yolks results from caged hens being fed things they don't normally eat, like cornmeal. Hens that are allowed to graze naturally eat a variety of grasses and produce naturally healthy eggs. Their diets are supplemented by feed consisting of flaxseed, which is rich in omega-3s. Several brands that mention "omega-3s" prominently on the label are available in health food stores and many supermarkets, and you can find out more about them by searching for omega-3 eggs on the Internet.

## IF YOU MUST EAT MEAT

Red meat is about the last thing you should eat in large quantities if you want to avoid inflammation and keep your weight down, as it is often loaded with omega-6 fatty acids. As with grains, the meat our ancestors ate was much more nutritious and less fattening than what we have been taught to eat. The early humans are believed to have gotten most of their nutrition from meat, fish, and shellfish, but the game they ate was wild and far leaner than most commercially available meat is now. Even the beef from grass-fed cattle of a hundred years ago was less deleterious to health than what comes from today's steers fattened on grain and shot full of antibiotics and hormones. So if you do need to eat red meat, there are a few ways you can stack the odds more in your favor. Organic, grass-fed beef, buffalo (bison), and lamb are available in most markets, although they're considerably more expensive than the other kind. Wild game, including venison and elk, are good sources of lean meat as well. Game birds such as turkey, pheasant, and grouse are other alternatives. Anything wild is more likely to be lean because it hasn't been fed grains specifically to increase weight and fat (purportedly to improve flavor) and has led a more active life.

## FOOD ALLERGIES

Foods that do not agree with us tend to cause allergic reactions and can produce compounds that interfere with normal body function while slowing down the healing of inflamed tissues.

These kinds of reactions are not in the same league as pollen allergies like hay fever, but they do involve the immune system and can exacerbate feelings of discomfort. The underlying problem is often one of faulty digestion or excessive consumption of specific foods. The most common allergenic foods are milk and dairy products, wheat, corn, eggs, beef, yeast, and soy. Even healthful foods can cause problems if you eat too much of them over a long period of time. Blood tests or elimination diets can help determine which foods you are allergic to, if any. Elimination diets require avoiding specific foods or food groups completely for a period of at least six months, then gradually adding them back into the diet and recording whether they create adverse reactions. It's a somewhat painstaking process but may be necessary to rule out the possibility that food allergies are contributing to your arthritis pain. Talk to your doctor about exploring this possibility.

## A TO Z:
## THE MOST HIGHLY RECOMMENDED FOODS

**Almonds** are high in monounsaturated fats (the same type of health-promoting fats found in olive oil), dietary fiber, and vitamin E, all valuable inflammation fighters. Because almonds are sweet and filling, especially in the form of pure almond butter, they make a healthier snack than most high-carbohydrate treats.

**Apples** are one of the most all-around helpful foods you can eat. They are high in both soluble and insoluble fiber, a combination that helps to reduce serum cholesterol. The pectin in apples absorbs excess water in the intestinal tract and helps to both soften and solidify the stool, aiding in elimination. The flavonoid quercetin, which apples have in quantity, has been strongly linked to reduced risk of heart disease.

**Apricots** are loaded with beta-carotene and fiber, and fresh apricots have a plentiful supply of vitamins A and C. Like most fruits, these delicious treats not only help reduce inflammation but also help prevent macular degeneration, which leads to impaired vision. Be careful about eating dried fruit, especially apricots, as they have much more sugar than the fresh variety. The pioneering nutritionist Bernard Jensen recommends soaking dried fruit in boiling water to dissolve residual sugar and then letting it reconstitute overnight.

**Avocados**, at 25 percent fruit oil, have the highest oil levels of all fruits. (The avocado is considered a fruit, not a vegetable, because of its large pit.) But like olive oil, the avocado is rich in oleic acid, the monounsaturated fat that is believed to help lower cholesterol. Some research has found compounds in avocados that kill cancer cells. The avocado is also an example of useful fat: Because valuable carotenoids in many other vegetables are fat-soluble, eating them with even a small amount of avocado makes their carotenoids more available to your body.

**Bananas** are high in vitamin $B_6$, potassium, and iron. The FDA has endorsed the value of potassium: "Diets containing foods that are good sources of potassium and low in sodium may reduce the risk of high blood pressure and stroke." One study of over 40,000 American male health professionals over four years determined that men who ate diets higher in potassium-rich foods had a substantially reduced risk of stroke. They also help with weight loss because they are rich in fiber, low in fat, and quite filling, and they feed the natural acidophilus bacteria in the intestines, necessary for proper digestion. What more could you ask from a delicious fruit that comes in its own wrapper?

**Beans** are an extraordinarily good deal in almost every aspect of nutrition. They are a fine source of protein, which can help replace body proteins broken down by inflammation. When combined with a whole grain like brown rice, beans form a complete protein chain comparable to those found in most meat. But they are far lower in calories (and cost) and very high in both soluble and insoluble fiber. Indeed, some cultures have been known to thrive on a diet consisting largely of beans and rice. Their good levels of iron can also help make up for the minor chronic blood loss from long-term NSAID or aspirin use. All beans are rich in antioxidants, but the deeper and darker their color, the more they possess. Thus black beans are your best bet; dollar for dollar and pound for pound, they are one of the best nutritional bargains you can find.

**Berries** are good sources of fiber, vitamin C, calcium, iron, potassium, and folic acid, and individual varieties each have special values. **Blueberries** are loaded with antioxidant phytonutrients called anthocyanidins and were rated the highest among sixty fruits and vegetables by researchers at Tufts University for their capacity to destroy free radicals. They are also high in vitamin C, manganese, and fiber and can help to heal both diarrhea and constipation. A slew of recent studies has confirmed the long-held anecdotal belief that **cranberries** can both treat and prevent urinary tract infections. As few as 2 cups of cranberry juice a day is all it takes. (But avoid cranberry juice cocktail which, like almost all juice drinks, is high in added sugar.) **Strawberries** are especially rich in anti-inflammatory properties, with phenols that decrease the activity of the COX enzyme, a job usually left for aspirin or ibuprofen, which can also cause intestinal bleeding. The tiny seeds on the outside that give the fruit its characteristic look also add to its high fiber content. And **raspberries** have several antioxidant flavonoids that can counteract bacteria and fungi, including *Candida*, which can lead to vaginal infections and irritable bowel syndrome.

**Broccoli** (and **broccoli rabe**) is already known for its anti-cancer properties, but it is also high in vitamins A and C, which protect the body against inflammation. A single cup of broccoli provides more than twice the recommended daily amount of vitamin C. Broccoli also contains glutathione, a powerful antioxidant and detoxifying agent that helps vitamins C and E do their job; glutathione is present in asparagus, cabbage, cauliflower, potatoes, tomatoes, grapefruit, peaches, and watermelon. The less you cook broccoli, the more chlorophyll remains to help prevent gas. Broccoli rabe, long a favorite of Italian immigrants in this country, is a slightly bitter, more flavorful variant that has many of the same nutrients as broccoli.

**Cabbage** is in the same genus (*Brassica*) as broccoli, cauliflower, kohlrabi, mustard greens, and Brussels sprouts, and is one of the most healing foods we have, especially for peptic ulcers. (The *Brassica* vegetables have been associated in studies with reduced risk of colon and breast cancer.) Like broccoli, cabbage is rich in vitamins C, $B_1$, $B_2$, and $B_6$, folate, and omega-3 fatty acids. All the vegetables in this family have strong anti-inflammatory properties.

**Cantaloupe** and other melons have vitamins A, B, and C and are potent thirst quenchers in the summer months. Some nutritionists recommend eating melon alone rather than in conjunction with other foods, but cantaloupe is so rich in nutrients, it's virtually a meal in itself. It's a good source of potassium, dietary fiber, folate, and vitamins $B_3$ and $B_6$. This combination of B complex vitamins and fiber helps the cells process carbohydrates, while ensuring that their sugars are delivered into the bloodstream gradually, keeping blood sugar regulated.

**Carrots** are not only high in vitamin A but are also loaded with beta-carotene, which helps fight inflammation. A fat-soluble antioxidant, beta-carotene, along with other carotenoids such as lutein and lycopene (found in tomatoes and watermelon), may also lower levels of deleterious C-reactive protein, although no definitive study has proven this. What *has* been shown is that consumption of fruits and vegetables rich in carotenoids and other nutrients *does* fight inflammation and tends to lower CRP levels.

**Celery** is high in sodium, which helps neutralize acids in the body, and compounds called pthalides, which relax the arterial muscles that regulate blood pressure. Pthalides also reduce stress hormones, one of whose effects is to cause blood vessels to constrict, and celery has been shown in several studies to lower both blood pressure and cholesterol.

**Collard greens, kale**, and **Swiss chard** are all high in calcium, and the calcium in kale is more readily assimilated than that in dairy products! Kale and chard come in a variety of colors, including red and purple, which are just as beneficial as the familiar dark green versions. Kale is especially noteworthy because, in addition to high levels of vitamins A and C, it contains omega-3 fatty acids and sulforaphane, a potent phytonutrient also found in collards and cabbage that boosts enzymes that detoxify cancer-causing chemicals. Sulforaphane has also been shown in a recent *Journal of Nutrition* study to help stop the spread of breast cancer cells, even in the later stages of their growth.

**Flaxseed** and **flaxseed oil** are rich in alpha linolenic acid, a precursor to the form of omega-3 called EPA, which is one of the most potent anti-inflammatory substances available, found also in fatty cold-water fish. Use flaxseed oil in salads or in fruit smoothies, but never cook with it, as it has a tendency to oxidize when heated. The seeds are hard to assimilate unless they are crushed or ground into oil.

**Ginger** is derived from the underground rhizome of a plant native to South Asia and is one of the world's oldest, best-known, and most versatile medicinal foods. It has been used for centuries in massage oil in Japan and in tea for coughs in China, and it is one of the best natural anti-nausea agents. Modern medicine is now recognizing some of ginger's time-honored virtues, especially for arthritis patients who want to decrease pain and protect their joints. Ginger's anti-inflammatory properties have been strongly supported by a number of scientific studies, most recently a yearlong double-blind study published in the November 2003 issue of *Osteoarthritis Cartilage*, in which participants who took ginger rather than a placebo experienced substantial relief from the pain and swelling of knee arthritis.

**Grapes** are rich in manganese, but their real value comes from their flavonoids, which give the purple color to grapes, grape juice, and red wine. Resveratrol, a phytoestrogen (or plant-derived, nonsteroidal compound), is present in the skins of grapes, in mulberries, nuts, wine, and other foods. The stronger the color of the grapes, the higher the concentration of resveratrol. The resveratrol present in red wine has been credited with explaining why the French, who traditionally have eaten high-fat diets, experience a lower incidence of heart disease and stroke than Americans. Red wine is also a blood thinner, and in moderation has been recommended for heart health. (Alcohol itself, however, is a liver toxin and, in forms including spirits and beer that lack red wine's high antioxidant content, is not recommended. White wine and white or green grapes have much less of an antioxidant effect than red wine and darker-colored grapes.) Studies have shown that resveratrol blocks the COX-2 gene from being activated and inactivates the enzyme created by that gene. Some believe that resveratrol may turn out to be better than aspirin in fighting diseases associated with COX-2, such as arthritis.

**Green tea** is the least processed form of true tea (as opposed to herbal teas) and so contains the most antioxidant polyphenols, especially a catechin called epigallo-catechin gallate (EGCG) that inhibits the expression of the interleukin-8 gene, a key to the arthritis inflammatory response. (Besides inhibiting the growth of cancer cells, EGCG kills cancer cells without harming healthy tissue.) Catechins have been found to be more potent free-radical scavengers than even vitamins C and E. One 2002 study reported that men and women who drank tea over a period of years had increased levels of bone density in certain joints. Researchers concluded that drinking tea regularly for at least ten years could boost bone mineral density by as much as five percent. In studies carried out in both Japan, where green tea is extremely popular, and the U.S., it has been found helpful in combating bacterial or viral infections (including tooth decay and bad breath) as well as chronic degenerative conditions such as periodontal disease and osteoporosis. A study by Western Reserve University in Cleveland concluded that drinking 4 or more cups of green tea a day could help prevent rheumatoid arthritis or reduce symptoms in individuals already suffering from the disease. As if that wasn't enough reason to drink this subtly delicious beverage, the catechins in green tea help thin the blood and prevent the formation of blood clots by blocking pro-inflammatory compounds derived from omega-6 fatty acids, specifically arachidonic acid, from which the inflammatory prostaglandin $D_2$ is derived.

**Kiwi fruit** is rich in vitamin C, the primary water-soluble antioxidant in the body, neutralizing free radicals that can cause damage to cells and lead to inflammation. But kiwi is also a good source of two of the most important fat-soluble antioxidants, vitamins E and A. By supplying us with fat- and water-soluble antioxidants, kiwi offers free-radical protection on all fronts.

**Olive oil** should be high on your list of arthritis-friendly foods. The Mediterranean Diet, which has proven successful in controlling weight and is considered heart-friendly, makes ample use of olive oil. This beneficial oil is high in monounsaturated omega-9 fatty acids (mainly oleic acid) and antioxidants. Studies have shown that olive oil offers protection against heart disease by controlling LDL cholesterol levels while raising HDL levels. It appears to decrease inflammation, and it is believed to have a beneficial effect on ulcers and gastritis. The Arthritis Foundation reports that researchers at the University of Athens Medical School found that people who consumed the most olive oil—about 3 tablespoons a day—were less likely than those with the lowest consumption to develop rheumatoid arthritis.

Be sure to buy primarily extra virgin olive oil, from the first cold pressing of the olives. This oil is the closest to natural olive oil because it is not heated in processing and, as a result, contains higher levels of antioxidants, particularly phenols and vitamin E, which protect DNA and genes from free-radical damage. It is the best alternative to corn and sunflower oils because it does not upset the critical omega-6 to omega-3 ratio. Be sure to store it in a cool, dark place, away from heat and sunlight to avoid rancidity.

**Onions** are in the same family as garlic, and all indications are that they help maintain low blood-sugar levels in the body. They also have an abundance of chromium, a trace mineral present in the molecule that helps cells respond appropriately to insulin. If you are sensitive to onions, eat them with parsley to moderate their effect on the stomach.

**Oranges** not only are ripe with vitamin C but also contain the flavanone herperidin, which has lowered cholesterol in some animal studies and has strong anti-inflammatory properties. But most of this phytonutrient is in the peel and inner white pith, so when you peel the orange, leave plenty of the soft white skin on. One study published in *Annals of the Rheumatic Diseases* in 2004 followed more than 23,000 men and women in the UK and showed that foods such as oranges that are rich in vitamin C provide protection against inflammatory polyarthritis, a form of rheumatoid arthritis involving two or more joints. Subjects who consumed the lowest amounts of vitamin C foods were more than three times as likely to develop arthritis as those who ate the highest amounts.

**Papaya** is rich in carotenes, vitamin C, flavonoids, B vitamins, folate and pantothenic acid, potassium, magnesium, and fiber. It also contains papain, a digestive enzyme used to treat sports injuries and allergies. Dried papaya is an excellent after-meal treat, as long as it is unsulfured.

**Pineapple** is rich in bromelain, a group of sulfur-containing, protein-digesting enzymes that diminish inflammation. In clinical trials, bromelain has reduced swelling in people suffering from acute sinusitis, sore throat, arthritis, and gout. To maximize bromelain's anti-inflammatory effects, eat pineapple by itself between meals so that its enzymes are not diverted to digesting food.

**Potatoes** have gotten a bad rap, nutritionally speaking. They are nightshade plants, and if you are sensitive to nightshades, of course you should avoid them. But if you steer clear of the deep-fried or sour-cream-stuffed variety, they are low in calories for the amount of fiber they provide.

**Sweet potatoes** are a good source of vitamins A and C, potent antioxidants with anti-inflammatory properties. They also have high amounts of vitamin $B_6$, which is needed by the body to break down homocysteine, a toxic amino acid that can directly damage blood vessel walls. Some people with normal or low cholesterol levels who nonetheless suffer a heart attack are often found to have high levels of homocysteine. To top it off, sweet potatoes, and their relative the yam, are pleasantly sweet. With a little maple syrup drizzled on top, they are as satisfying as most desserts and may help control weight.

**Tofu** is a fine source of protein that is made from the curds of soybean milk and is a staple of any vegetarian diet. It's packed with manganese, iron, and tryptophan and can also help to lower total cholesterol levels by as much as 30 percent and to control levels of triglycerides in the blood. Triglycerides are the form in which fat is carried in the blood and stored in the body, and an excess of them has been linked to the occurrence of coronary artery disease in some people.

**Tomatoes** are a nightshade food, but they should not be eliminated lightly from the diet. They are a major source of the carotenoid lycopene, which has been studied extensively in humans and found to protect cells and other structures in the body from oxygen damage. Tomatoes have also been linked to protecting DNA inside white blood cells and, according to one Finnish study, helping to prevent heart disease and stroke, as well as a variety of cancers, including prostate, breast, colorectal, and pancreatic.

**Turmeric,** a popular spice that is a relative of the ginger plant, has been used in Ayurvedic and traditional Chinese medicine to treat blood disorders and liver problems, and is known to serve as a powerful COX-2 inhibitor, with none of the side effects of the pharmaceutical COX-2 drugs. One component of turmeric, the powerful anti-inflammatory chemical curcumin, is said to be 50 percent as effective as cortisone, stimulating the body's cortisone-like chemicals without the danger or expense. But the amount of curcumin in turmeric isn't enough to have an anti-inflammatory effect on its own, so you might do better with a daily dose of 500 to 1,000 mg standardized to 95 percent curcuminoids.

**Water,** especially **mineral water,** is one of the most nutritious, arthritis-friendly drinks you can consume. For one thing, dehydration can exacerbate the pain caused by arthritis. When you don't drink enough water, inflammation becomes worse, so be careful to drink at least 60 to 80 ounces of water every day—that's eight to ten 8-ounce glasses, or about 2 quarts. Caffeine and alcohol contain diuretics that cause the body to lose more water, so drink them in moderation. If you have more than a couple of alcoholic drinks at night, be sure to drink several glasses of water before retiring. Mineral water has the added benefit of containing valuable nutrients. And all pure water contains no calories, so it is the perfect drink.

**Whole grain** is the only form in which you should consume wheat, rice, barley, millet, and other grains. Most commercially produced breads, pastas, noodles, and baked goods in the United States are made with bleached white flour that has been processed into what is called "60 percent extraction." In this procedure, 40 percent of the original wheat grain is removed, including the most nutritious parts, the bran and germ, along with over half of the vitamins $B_1$, $B_2$, $B_3$, and E, folic acid, calcium, phosphorus, zinc, copper, iron, and fiber. As a result, in the last century the government required enrichment of processed wheat flour with vitamins $B_1$, $B_2$, and $B_3$, and iron, but this still does not replace as much of these nutrients as is removed. To get the greatest value from grains, you should use only unbleached flour for baking. Avoid packaged breads and pastas that have "enriched" flour or long lists of chemicals on the label. If you put a loaf of bread in your breadbox and it doesn't form mold in a couple of days, it's probably not made with whole grains.

Don't limit yourself to just the usual wheat and rice, but vary the menu with barley, buckwheat, millet, spelt, and quinoa, each of which has distinctive nutritional qualities. Quinoa (pronounced KEEN-wah) is not actually a grain; it is the seed of a leafy plant that is a distant cousin of spinach. Cultivated in the Andes and once called the gold of the Incas, quinoa has excellent reserves of protein. Unlike other grains, it is not missing the amino acid lysine, so its protein is more complete and has been rated as equivalent to that in milk. Rich in iron, quinoa also has high levels of potassium and B vitamins and is a good source of magnesium, zinc, copper, and manganese. Other grains, such as buckwheat and brown rice, are rich in selenium, a trace mineral that has been shown to reduce the risk of colon cancer. And all grains are excellent sources of dietary fiber.

When shopping for whole-grain breads, beware of marketing ploys. Many commercial producers offer variations such as "wheat bread," which is essentially white bread with bits of wheat added to enhance color and texture but with no real gain in nutrition. Make sure the label says "whole wheat" or "whole grain wheat" and the list of ingredients says "100 percent whole wheat" and doesn't say "enriched flour." Mixed-grain breads are fine as long as the label says "whole grain." Dark rye bread is also nutritious and a good source of dietary fiber. The noncellulose polysaccharides in rye bread have a high water-binding capacity, which results in a feeling of fullness that can help you eat less. But commercial producers of genuine whole-grain breads and cereals may add sugar, high-fructose corn syrup, soybean oil, and other inflammatory ingredients loaded with omega-6, so check the ingredients carefully. Better yet, buy your breads, cereals, and baked goods in a health food store or the organic section of your local supermarket.

## EATING OUT

It's often a challenge to get a healthful meal when you go out to eat or are traveling. First, be sure to steer clear of fast food restaurants, as they all use a lot of unnecessary salt, sugar (even in French fries!), hydrogenated oils, and fats. Ethnic restaurants featuring Eastern cuisine are often a good deal, especially the lunch buffets you find at many Indian, Thai, Chinese, and Japanese eateries. They tend to use smaller portions of meat and fish; more vegetables and anti-inflammatory herbs like ginger, turmeric, and garlic; and as shorter cooking times. But be sure to ask if they use MSG (monosodium glutamate), a taste-enhancing chemical that can lead to headaches and other allergic reactions. In addition, some Chinese dishes made with extra sugar and many Indian and Thai specialties made with cream and/or coconut sauces can be highly caloric. Look for menu items featuring steamed vegetables, sautéed fish, and other items that are likely to be lower in calories. Remember that being overweight is a contributing cause of arthritis and arthritis pain, so anything you can do to reduce calories while eating more healthful meals will help you avoid the problems associated with arthritis.

Choose from one of the many typical takeout dishes below. These are based on the takeout menus from ethnic and other restaurants available in most cities and many towns.

- Chicken with broccoli
- Sautéed shrimp with ginger and garlic
- Bean curd with black mushrooms and garlic sauce
- Sautéed mustard greens, snow peas, zucchini, eggplant, or green beans
- Tandoori salmon with raita (cucumbers in plain yogurt)

- Sashimi (sushi without the rice: raw tuna, salmon, yellowtail, shrimp), served with radish, wasabi, and pickled ginger.
- Thai hot and sour soup with shrimp
- Veggie burger on whole-grain bun
- Greek salad (green leaf and romaine lettuce, artichoke hearts, cherry tomatoes, olives, cucumbers, feta cheese with vinaigrette dressing)
- Tuna fish wrap sandwich
- Grilled salmon steak with portobello mushrooms
- Curried egg salad on a bed of dark green lettuce
- Guacamole (avocado, tomatoes, onions, garlic, cilantro, hot pepper and lime juice)
- Gazpacho (cold soup made with tomatoes, cucumber, green pepper, celery, onion, garlic, lemon juice, and olive oil)
- Tuscan bean soup (made with cannellini or Great Northern beans, kale, green cabbage, Brussels sprouts, Swiss chard, leek, onion, carrot, celery, plum tomatoes, and whole-grain bread)

## SHOPPING LISTS

When you shop for groceries, it's a good idea to bring along a list of foods in each category that are inflammation fighters, as well as a list of foods to be sure to avoid. As I have already said, variety is the key to a diet with balanced levels of all nutrients. However, if you don't have time to shop selectively on any given day, you would do well to consider the following list of best bets, foods that tend to provide higher levels of nutrients while helping to fight inflammation and arthritis. When you have more time, copy three or four items from each boxed list and shop for them. Put a check mark next to the ones you bought. Try to purchase different varieties on future shopping days.

# BEST BETS

| Vegetables | Fruits | Fish | Other Meat and Poultry |
|---|---|---|---|
| Broccoli | Apples | Salmon | Grass-fed beef |
| Kale | Blackberries | Sardines | Organic lamb |
| Spinach | Kiwi | Tuna | Skinless chicken breast |

# SHOPPING LISTS

| Vegetables | | Fruits | |
|---|---|---|---|
| Asparagus | Garlic | Apples | Papayas |
| Bell peppers (green, | Green beans | Apricots | Pineapple |
| red, yellow) | Kale (red, green, | Avocados | Plums |
| Broccoli, broccoli | black) | Bananas | Prunes |
| rabe | Lettuce (romaine, | Blackberries | Raisins |
| Brussels sprouts | red or green | Blueberries | Strawberries |
| Cabbage (green, | leaf) | Cantaloupe | Watermelon |
| purple) | Mushrooms | Cranberries | |
| Cauliflower | (portobello) | Grapefruit | |
| Celery | Mustard greens | Grapes | |
| Chard (Swiss, red, | Onions (red, yellow) | Honeydew melon | |
| rainbow) | Scallions | Kiwi fruit | |
| Collard greens | Spinach | Lemons | |
| Cucumber | Squash (winter, | Limes | |
| Eggplant (black, | summer) | Mangoes | |
| white, pink) | | Oranges | |

| Whole Grains | Nuts and Seeds | Beans and Legumes |
|---|---|---|
| Barley | Almonds | Black beans |
| Brown rice | Cashews | Cannellini beans |
| Buckwheat cereal | Flaxseed | Garbanzo beans |
| Corn bread | Pumpkin seeds | Great Northern beans |
| Millet | Sesame seeds | Kidney beans |
| Oats (oatmeal) | Sunflower seeds | Lentils (red, green) |
| Quinoa | Walnuts (black, English) | Navy beans |
| Rye bread | | Pinto beans |
| Spelt cake | | Soybeans (miso, soymilk) |
| Whole wheat bread | | Tempeh |
| | | Tofu |

| Herbs and Spices | Dairy | Oils |
|---|---|---|
| Basil | Goat cheese | Borage oil |
| Black pepper | Low-fat cheese | Flaxseed oil |
| Cayenne pepper | Low-fat milk (Use | Olive oil |
| Chili pepper | soymilk as substitute | |
| Cinnamon | whenever possible) | |
| Cloves | Low-fat yogurt | |
| Coriander | Omega-3 eggs | |
| Cumin | | |
| Dill weed | | |
| Ginger | | |
| Oregano | | |
| Peppermint | | |
| Rosemary | | |
| Sage | | |
| Thyme | | |
| Turmeric | | |

# CHAPTER SIX

# THE ARTHRITIS Rx NUTRITIONAL SUPPLEMENT AND OTHER SUPPLEMENTS

In most cases, a nutritionally balanced diet is the first line of defense against arthritis. But because of a variety of factors, including the depletion of the soil and the farming practices of the large agribusiness corporations that have taken over growing the majority of crops, much of the food available in American supermarkets is lacking in the vital nutrients needed to keep arthritis and other diseases at bay. In addition, some individuals need to follow highly restricted diets because of other health conditions, or they simply don't have the time, or the will, to eat properly. Even those who do take care with their diets may not always be certain of getting enough of the vitamins, minerals, and nutrients they need. Thus, they turn to nutritional supplements. The supplement market has grown to astonishing proportions in the past decade or so, and although it now accounts for billions of dollars in annual sales, quality standards are still largely unregulated. Yet in my own experience as a physician, supplements have been proven to have enormous value to many people suffering from arthritis. If you choose carefully from the many supplements on the market that have been independently evaluated, you can make improvements in your ability to control pain and slow the progress of arthritis.

Because of the positive results in scientifically sound studies, I often suggest that my patients take a mixture of glucosamine, chondroitin sulfate, and ginger. To make it easy for them to do so, I have come up with an Arthritis Rx nutritional supplement, Zingerflex, which includes 1,500 mg of glucosamine, 1,200 mg of chondroitin sulfate, and 510 mg of ginger. It is available at zingerflex.com.

Why that combination? As people age, their bodies lose the ability to produce sufficient glucosamine, a natural substance found in cartilage. This may in turn make the joint susceptible to inflammation that leads to pain, limited mobility, and other symptoms of arthritis. Chondroitin sulfate, a substance found in human and animal cartilage, is often used to protect joints. Chondroitin sulfate not only inhibits the activity of enzymes that break down the cartilage, but is also believed to stimulate the production of glycosaminoglycans, which are the building blocks of cartilage. Chondroitin sulfate is made from cow, fish, and pork cartilage. It comes as a pill, powder, and liquid. The supplement form of glucosamine is derived from crab shells. Some individuals can't use chondroitin sulfate and glucosamine, because they can cause stomach upset, bloating, and other GI side effects. **Anyone who is allergic to shellfish must avoid glucosamine.**

These supplements have gained great popularity in recent years among people seeking to alleviate the pain of arthritis. The public buys more glucosamine ($6 billion per year) than all of the anti-inflammatories combined. More than fifteen controlled studies have shown that the supplements may reduce pain. One study in the British medical journal *The Lancet* found that glucosamine may also slow the rate at which cartilage is worn away. The results of a well-designed study by the National Institutes of Health (NIH) begun in 2002 provide important guidelines. Called the Glucosamine/Chondroitin Arthritis Intervention Trial (GAIT), the study enrolled 1,588 patients at thirteen study sites. It used standardized products and doses and was designed to measure changes in joint space, a means of evaluating whether the supplements have an impact on cartilage. The GAIT trial data presented at the American College of Rheumatology meeting in November 2005 in San Diego concluded that the combination of 1,500 mg of glucosamine and 1,200 mg of chondroitin sulfate as a supplement taken daily was at least as effective as the anti-inflammatory Celebrex in treating knee arthritis. They concluded that the combination of glucosamine and chondroitin sulfate is effective in treating moderate to severe knee pain due to osteoarthritis. At the same meeting, the large European multicenter trial called GUIDE concluded that 1,500 mg of glucosamine sulfate a day was superior to 3,000 mg of acetaminophen (Tylenol) taken daily to reduce pain from knee osteoarthritis. They determined that glucosamine sulfate may be the preferred symptomatic medication in knee osteoarthritis. These two large, well-conducted trials demonstrate that 1,500 mg of glucosamine combined with 1,200 mg of chondroitin sulfate is well tolerated and is effective in treating moderate to severe knee pain due to osteoarthritis.

Much has been written about the efficacy of glucosamine and chondroitin sulfate as treatments for arthritis, but less attention has been paid to a much older remedy that is a commonly used spice in Asian cooking. Derived from the underground stem of a plant native to South Asia, ginger is one of the world's oldest, best-known, and most versatile medicinal foods.

In the clinical trial of 250 patients in 2001, published in *Arthritis & Rheumatism*, researchers at the University of Miami Medical School found that ginger was as effective as conventional painkillers in controlling arthritis pain. Some participants took 255 mg of ginger twice a day; the others received a placebo. After six weeks, two-thirds of those who received the ginger pills reported significantly more relief than those taking the placebo. The researchers stressed that the effect was similar to that seen with trials using conventional drugs. They believe that the positive results occurred because ginger possesses a biochemical structure similar to non-steroidal drugs such as aspirin, an important inflammation fighter. It even contains a flavonoid that serves as a mild COX-2 inhibitor.

An earlier study in Denmark by Prof. Krishna Srivastava, Ph.D., of Odense University had found that 55 percent of arthritis patients and 74 percent of those who had rheumatoid arthritis who took 5 grams of fresh ginger or 1 gram (1,000 mg) of powdered ginger daily for six weeks also reported "marked relief from pain." Prof.

Srivastava as well as scientists at the University of Miami Medical School have stressed that more research is required to explore fully the role of ginger in managing arthritis symptoms.

Getting ginger into the diet is easy. Fresh ginger is available in the produce department of most supermarkets and health food stores. Several teaspoons of grated fresh ginger can be added to batter for muffins, steamed vegetables, and salad dressings. A few drops of ginger juice can be used in hot or cold beverages. Some foods already contain ginger, such as ginger herbal teas and cold drinks and gingersnaps. And many international cuisines, such as Thai, Indian, Chinese, and Japanese food, incorporate fresh or pickled ginger into their meals. But since it's not easy to consume 510 mg of ginger daily, the Zingerflex supplement is a good backup. Some individuals, however, must be wary of consuming ginger. Those who take anticoagulants should consult their physicians before using ginger, as it can thin the blood.

In addition to the Zingerflex supplement, only one other commercially available product is independently tested for purity. Cosamine DS contains glucosamine and chondroitin sulfate in the same ratio as Zingerflex but includes manganese ascorbate rather than ginger as a third ingredient. A separate product created by Dr. Andrew Weil called Zyflamend promises to help reduce inflammation with natural herbs. It includes a blend of ginger, turmeric, green tea, holy basil, and rosemary, among other ingredients. Apart from ginger and green tea, however, most of these ingredients have not been shown in clinical trials to relieve inflammation and arthritis pain. Nonetheless, several patients of mine have reported good results from using this product, and I find nothing dangerous in it.

## THUMBS UP FOR SUPPLEMENTS

A sixty-two-year-old business executive named Bill came to see me complaining of arthritis of the thumb. He had a genetic predisposition to hand arthritis, as his mother had had similar problems, and in his case the pain was significant. Bill had lost his ability to tolerate anti-inflammatories and had been told by a hand surgeon that he needed to have surgery on his thumb. He was coming to me for a second opinion.

Because Bill didn't seem to have any advanced damage to the cartilage in his hand, I decided to start him off on nutritional supplements. I gave him the Zinger-flex supplement and also had him squeeze a sponge in a water bucket one hundred times every day and ice the thumb at night. As a result of these simple processes, Bill became pain-free, regained full range of motion in his thumb, and did not need to have surgery. Although nobody had ever mentioned the possibility of taking supplements before, Bill now swears by them.

## MSM AND SAMe

Two other supplements have been used by some individuals with arthritis: MSM (methylsulfonylmethane), an organic sulfur compound found naturally in fruits, vegetables, and grains; and SAMe (S-adenosyl-L-methionine), a naturally occurring chemical in the body. I do not recommend these supplements for my patients, however, because research on MSM has been limited to a few animal studies. One small study with people showed that it may ease pain, but there is no evidence at this time that MSM is safe and effective. Most of the research concerning the efficacy of SAMe has been done in Europe. Studies there suggest that SAMe treats pain and stiffness in the same way that the non-steroidal anti-inflammatory drugs (NSAIDs) do, but that SAMe produces fewer GI side effects. However, I believe that more long-term clinical trials with both these supplements must be done before physicians can recommend them.

Although supplements can be purchased over the counter in grocery stores, health food stores, on the Internet, and through other outlets, they should be used cautiously. Because they are not directly regulated by the Food and Drug Administration the way prescription medications are, there is no way to determine whether the products contain the amount or type of supplement listed on their labels. Therefore, make sure that any supplement you take is tested for purity by an independent laboratory. One way to do this is to look for "GMP" on the label. GMP refers to the Good Manufacturing Practice, a set of regulations promulgated by the FDA under the authority of the Federal Food, Drug, and Cosmetic Act (Chapter IV for food; Chapter V, subchapters A, B, C, D, and E for drugs and devices). These regulations, which have the force of law, require that manufacturers, processors, and packagers of drugs, medical devices, and some nutritional supplements ensure that their products are safe, pure, and effective, and minimize or eliminate instances of contamination and errors. Applied to nutritional supplements, the GMP emblem ensures that a supplement meets the standards for strength, purity, and the rate at which it dissolves in the system, as well as assuring a hygienic manufacturing process, as with the Zingerflex supplement.

# CHAPTER SEVEN

# THE ARTHRITIS Rx PLAN:
# A WEEKLY SAMPLER

Now that I have explained all the elements for treating and reducing arthritis pain, it's time to put them together into a simple, comprehensive plan of action. In this chapter I lay out a one-week sample plan designed to be practical but effective. The Arthritis Rx Plan incorporates the Arthritis Rx Exercises, the Zingerflex supplement, and the Arthritis Rx Diet, yet it requires a minimal commitment of your time.

You should notice minor improvements on a daily basis, but the full benefits of this plan begin to take effect after about eight weeks. You may experience mildly increased discomfort during the first two to three weeks of the plan, but that is absolutely normal, since you are altering ingrained habits to which your body has grown accustomed. If there is any severe increase in discomfort, however, you should seek the advice of a physician.

For maximum benefit, you should take daily four capsules of the Zingerflex supplement. Take two in the morning with breakfast, and two more with lunch.

You may, of course, take any other supplements, as long as they add up to a daily total of 1,500 mg of glucosamine, 1,200 mg of chondroitin sulfate, and 510 mg of ginger. Again, anyone with diabetes or compromised kidney function, or on blood thinners should seek the advice of a physician before taking this supplement. Make sure that the supplements you are taking are GMP certified and independently tested for purity.

The daily exercises in my plan are arthritis-friendly and are meant to minimize impact and high-shear stresses on the joints while restoring flexibility, strength, endurance, and aerobic fitness. You will alternate days on which you do the Arthritis Rx Exercises with days on which you do some other form of mildly aerobic exercise that is arthritis-friendly. These include walking, aquatherapy, and use of the elliptical trainer or recumbent bicycle. You will be doing twenty to thirty minutes of exercise each day. You do not necessarily have to progress from Arthritis Rx Series A to Series B or C unless you are completely comfortable and pain-free.

## DAILY STAPLES

The diet portion of the plan offers a recipe for at least one meal a day for you to incorporate but offers guidelines for creating any number of breakfast, lunch, and dinner menus that you can mix and match. Over a period of weeks, you can develop your own recipes based on the use of the anti-inflammatory foods discussed in Chapter Five. (For convenience, all the recipes appear in alphabetical order at the end of this chapter.) It's also useful to develop a few daily standbys—simple meals that you can add to for variety, as long as the ingredients are anti-inflammatory. Breakfast, for example, can be a problem for many people. A lot of us think it's great to have a Danish and coffee or pancakes every day. But if you're going to get into a habit, at least make it a good one. Two eggs made into a vegetable omelet or scrambled with onions and greens is one staple breakfast that you can vary infinitely or keep the same without sacrificing nutrition. Two eggs supply about 40 percent of the 50 grams of protein you need every day but only 136 calories. (If you use eggs from free-range hens, especially those that are rich in omega-3, you can increase the beneficial effects.) Mix in ¼ to ½ cup of cooked kale, spinach, or another green. (You can use frozen spinach or kale as long as no undesirable ingredients, such as corn oil, MSG, or sugar, are listed on the package. Canned greens should be avoided.) If you like, you can slice up 1½ ounces of chicken or turkey sausage, with no nitrites, for added protein and only a slight calorie boost (half a 3-ounce link is about 75 calories but adds another 8 grams of protein). Cooking with olive oil eliminates the need for butter or vegetable oils. Get a small mister or spray diffuser and fill it with extra virgin olive oil, then spray on enough to coat your skillet lightly before cooking. (See recipes for details.) Or use a non-fat cooking spray such as PAM, which comes in an olive oil variety. There is some evidence that exposing egg yolks to oxygen while cooking them at high heat—say, by scrambling them—may be less healthful than poaching or boiling. So you may want to vary how you cook your eggs, occasionally frying them over easy (using olive oil, not butter), poaching them, or having hard- or soft-boiled eggs. Boiling half a dozen eggs in advance and storing them in the refrigerator is a great convenience if you don't always have time to cook in the morning.

## SALAD DAYS

Just as it's helpful to have a breakfast staple that you can fall back on in the mornings, a lunch staple can ensure that you eat a decent meal at midday even if you don't have much time. Your best bet most days is a simple salad. It may be simple in terms of preparation time, but it will still contain a diverse array of vitamins, minerals, and nutrients that you'll be able to pack into that salad with surprisingly little effort. Start with a few basic ingredients and add as much or as little as you want, based on what's in season and readily available. Most gourmet chefs agree that the secret to fine cuisine isn't necessarily the time of preparation or the sophistication of the cooking implements you use but the quality of your ingredients. If the ingredients of your salads are well chosen, fresh, and organic, not only will your salad taste better but it will leave your body better equipped to fight inflammation and the pain of arthritis.

Few summer salads are more refreshing than one made with tomatoes, red onions, and cucumbers, with a light balsamic vinaigrette dressing. If the tomatoes are ripe (heirlooms are tastiest, but any plump tomato will do), and the onions and cucumbers are thinly sliced, you don't need a heavy, creamy dressing. You can make your own balsamic vinaigrette dressing (serves several salads) with ½ cup extra virgin olive oil, 1 teaspoon of balsamic or red wine vinegar, salt and pepper to taste, and 1 teaspoon Dijon mustard for spice. You can also buy vinaigrette at any good health food store (check the label to make sure it has no vegetable oil in it). It's a nice break from the usual green salad, although you can certainly add a bit of romaine or red leaf lettuce and sliced avocado. The secret is to let the tomatoes marinate for a while in the vinaigrette before adding the other ingredients and tossing.

Of course, you can start with lettuce, as long as you use anything but iceberg, a nutritionally worthless hybrid created in the early twentieth century to keep lettuce from spoiling when it was shipped to market. Then layer the ingredients by varying colors and textures. Purple cabbage shredded thinly adds color and crunch; celery ramps up the moisture level; sliced or shredded carrots, diced fennel bulb, bok choy, baby spinach, and mesclun greens all make fine additions. You can add special ingredients such as olives or artichoke hearts, but only in moderation. Be sure to check the caloric values first. As long as most of the ingredients are on the list of recommended foods, you should be all right. And with the abundance of salad bars and make-your-own stations in supermarkets, delis, and restaurants today, you can make salads a part of your daily diet without any preparation. (Just avoid the non-veggie add-ons like cheese cubes, bacon bits, biscuits, and croutons.)

In colder weather, summer salads may feel less refreshing, but you can make a warm salad from sliced roasted potatoes, cooked lentils, and a wide variety of steamed veggies, from beets to asparagus tips. To increase the protein count in any of these salads, just top them with grilled chicken breast, turkey, salmon, tuna, or shrimp.

Whatever you prepare, you can save time by making a large salad and refrigerating what you don't eat in an airtight container. Generally it will keep longer if you don't add dressing before serving, but one exception is the tomato and red onion salad I mentioned. The longer the tomatoes and other ingredients sit in the vinaigrette, the tastier they get. The beauty of balsamic vinegar is that just a few drops makes a tasty salad that isn't overly acidic.

## BE FRUIT-FULL

The most delicious part of any anti-inflammatory, arthritis-friendly diet is also the easiest to consume. You can eat fruit at any time of day, as part of a meal, as dessert, and alone as a healthful snack. It's easy enough to eat an apple, banana, peach, or plum by itself—and remember, that counts as one serving of the five or more servings of plant foods you need each day. If you have a little more time, you can slice up a few strawberries, add pineapple chunks (most stores sell pineapple already peeled and cored), a few red or purple grapes, blueberries, raspberries, or sliced kiwi fruit. Pour a little pure fruit juice over it and you have a royal treat loaded with antioxidants. Buy fresh fruit once a week and leave a few apples, bananas, plums, or apricots in a bowl to get your family in the habit of snacking on fruit. Refrigerate fruit that is ripe to preserve its life. But by all means avoid canned fruit, especially fruit cocktail with the mandatory maraschino cherry colored with red dye or fruit packaged in corn syrup. Some lines of frozen organic strawberries, blueberries, and cherries are acceptable substitutes, but as a rule, fresh fruit is best.

## EATING ON THE GO

I realize that you don't always have time to cook, especially breakfast and lunch, when you're in a hurry to get the kids off to school or to get to work. Here are a few suggestions for arthritis-friendly eating when you're on the go.

### Arthritis Rx Breakfast on the Go

- Whole-grain cereal without added sugar, such as Multi Grain Squares, 1 cup, with soymilk, or lowfat or fat-free milk
- Fat-free plain or fruit-flavored yogurt, 1 cup, with ½ cup sugar-free granola sprinkled on top (check the label)

### Arthritis Rx Lunch on the Go (can also be ordered as takeout)

- One 6-ounce can of tuna fish mixed with minced onion and 4 tablespoons of light mayonnaise, salt and pepper to taste, on whole wheat bread
- Veggie burger on whole wheat bread (condiments optional)

### Arthritis Rx Dessert on the Go

- Kiwi fruit, peeled, with blackberries (sliced strawberries optional), mixed with ¼ cup light whipping cream
- One apple cored and sliced, sprinkled with cinnamon and 1 tablespoon brown sugar. Microwave for about 2 minutes (microwave time may vary). Serving suggestion: add light whipping cream on top

There's a wise old rule of nutrition that is more valid than ever these days: Eat breakfast like a king (or queen); eat lunch like a prince (or a princess); and eat supper like a poor person. If you follow that rubric, your body will get the bulk of its nutrition when you need it most, during the workday. You will also have more time to digest the food and work off the calories, so you'll sleep better and control your weight at the same time. Most restaurants charge considerably less for many of the same dishes at lunchtime, making this a wise economic choice as well. And after eating a good-sized lunch, you may find that a simple soup and salad for dinner are enough to satisfy you.

Again, this may not always be practical, given the demands of the day, but the closer you can come to this formula, the better chance you'll have of controlling your weight and resisting the urge to snack on salty chips, cookies, or chocolates, or consume juice drinks and coffee for energy. Ideally, your energy should come from your food. I hope that you will be able to incorporate my recipes and menu suggestions into your daily regimen, combined with proper exercise and nutritional supplements to eliminate arthritis pain, enhance mobility, and slow the progression of arthritis. Here is a sample of a week's worth of diet and exercises to help you launch the Arthritis Rx Plan. You can find the recipes at the end of this chapter.

## MONDAY

| *Breakfast* | *Calories* |
| --- | --- |
| Breakfast veggie omelet (2 eggs) | 360 |
| Green tea and whole-grain toast with jam (1 slice) | 140 |

| *Lunch* | |
| --- | --- |
| Gazpacho, 1 cup | 200 |
| Open-faced turkey sandwich (3 slices) on 1 slice whole-grain bread | 400 |
| Sliced peaches | 100 |

| *Snack* | |
| --- | --- |
| Almonds (15) | 100 |

| *Dinner* | |
| --- | --- |
| Breast of chicken (8 oz.) with steamed broccoli | 400 |
| Green salad with avocado and sesame vinaigrette dressing | 300 |

**Exercise**

Arthritis Rx exercise regimen combined with two capsules twice a day (at breakfast and lunch) of the Arthritis Rx nutritional supplement Zingerflex, or the same ingredients with the same daily total. Start with Series A for a minimum of six weeks before moving on to Series B if you feel the need for an extra level of fitness. Do not start Series C unless you have full pain-free range of motion in the arthritic joint. The majority of arthritis patients do well maintaining the Series A exercises without ever moving on.

TUESDAY

| *Breakfast* | *Calories* |
|---|---|
| Oatmeal (1 cup) with soymilk | 300 |

| *Lunch* | |
|---|---|
| Romaine lettuce and tomato salad, choice of dressing | 285 |
| topped with sliced grilled chicken (2½ oz.) | 415 |

| *Snack* | |
|---|---|
| Organic protein bar | 200 |

| *Dinner* | |
|---|---|
| Roast chicken (8 oz.) w/spicy mango and strawberry chutney | 800 |

**Exercise**

Sixteen minutes of walking. If unable to tolerate walking, do sixteen minutes on the recumbent bicycle or elliptical trainer, or do aquatherapy the first week. Increase the time you spend exercising by two minutes per week so that at the end of the eight weeks you are doing thirty minutes a day. If you cannot tolerate thirty minutes, at least do physical exercise for twenty minutes daily. Combine with two Zingerflex pills twice during the day.

| Breakfast | Calories |
|---|---|
| 2 scrambled eggs w/onions and smoked salmon (2 oz.) | 350 |

| Lunch | |
|---|---|
| Tuna fish wrap sandwich with small green salad | 800 |

| Snack | |
|---|---|
| Strawberries (1 cup) w/light cream | 100 |

| Dinner | |
|---|---|
| Butternut squash soup (1 cup) | 200 |
| 2 slices whole-grain bread | 150 |
| Stir-fried shrimp (12 large) with sliced leeks and ginger | 300 |

## Exercise:

Arthritis Rx exercise regimen combined with two Zingerflex capsules twice a day.

THURSDAY

| Breakfast | Calories |
|---|---|
| Hot whole-grain cereal (1 ½ cups) with soymilk | 300 |
| Strawberries (1 cup) w/organic whipped cream or light cream | 145 |

| Lunch | |
|---|---|
| Grilled salmon steak (6 oz.) w/sautéed spinach | 400 |

| | |
|---|---|
| Low-fat plain yogurt (1 cup) and blueberries | 200 |

| *Dinner* | |
|---|---|
| Skinless chicken breast (4 oz.) | 200 |
| Ginger and garlic greens w/brown rice (1 cup) | 350 |

## Exercise:

Recumbent bicycle (substitute with an elliptical trainer if unable to tolerate the bicycle). Once again, start out with sixteen minutes and add two minutes every week so that by the end of eight weeks you are doing thirty minutes. If you cannot get up to thirty minutes, that is okay, but the minimal goal should be twenty minutes. Combine with two capsules of Zingerflex supplement twice a day.

FRIDAY

| *Breakfast* | *Calories* |
|---|---|
| 2 eggs over easy w/one link turkey sausage | 400 |
| 1 Ezekiel English muffin | 150 |

| *Lunch* | |
|---|---|
| Sautéed tofu (1 cup) w/black mushrooms | 600 |

| *Snack* | |
|---|---|
| Sliced apples w/granola sprinkle (1 oz.) | 200 |

| *Dinner* | |
|---|---|
| Tuna and grape tomatoes on brown rice | 680 |

**Exercise:**

Arthritis Rx exercise regimen combined with Zingerflex capsules twice daily.

SATURDAY

| Breakfast | Calories |
|---|---|
| Fat-free plain or fruit-flavored yogurt (1 cup) | 120 |
| Sugar-free granola (1 oz.) | 80 |

| Lunch | |
|---|---|
| Avocado sandwich spread on two slices of whole-grain bread | 700 |
| Raspberries (1 cup) w/organic whipped cream or light cream | 130 |

| Snack | |
|---|---|
| Organic blueberry pie | 200 |

| Dinner | |
|---|---|
| Tuscan bean soup | 700 |
| Sliced plums | 100 |

**Exercise:**

Walk on a soft, even surface such as clay, or a treadmill if possible, sixteen minutes the first week, and add two minutes a week till you have reached thirty minutes by eight weeks. Again, the goal here is to be able to walk a minimum of twenty minutes. If unable to tolerate walking, substitute aquatherapy in waist-high water. Combine with two Zingerflex pills twice daily.

| Breakfast | Calories |
|---|---|
| Whole wheat pancakes (3) with pure maple syrup and blueberries with organic whipped cream or light cream | 550 |

| Lunch | |
|---|---|
| Veggie burger on whole-grain bun w/soy mayonnaise | 500 |

| Snack | |
|---|---|
| Fruit cocktail: sliced banana, cherries, blueberries, pineapple | 200 |

| Dinner | |
|---|---|
| Ginger-garlic salmon fillet with steamed broccoli | 700 |

**Exercise**

Sunday is a rest day to let the musculoskeletal system recover. But be sure to continue to take two Zingerflex supplements twice daily.

# ARTHRITIS Rx RECIPES

---

## Avocado Sandwich Spread

INGREDIENTS

4 medium-sized Haas avocados

Juice of 1 lime

2 medium tomatoes, coarsely chopped

1 large red onion, roughly chopped

2 hot peppers (optional)

Salt to taste

Cut avocados in half lengthwise, cutting around the pit. Twist to separate the halves and scoop out the pit with a spoon, then use the spoon to scoop the avocados from their skin. Place the avocados in a bowl and mash with fork. Combine with lime juice, tomatoes, onion, peppers, and salt. Mash until smooth. Serve on whole wheat bread. Serves 4.

## Balsamic Vinaigrette Dressing

INGREDIENTS
½ cup extra virgin olive oil
1 tsp. balsamic vinegar or red wine vinegar
1 tsp. Dijon mustard
Freshly ground pepper
Salt to taste

Pour ingredients into a small jar and shake vigorously, or whisk in a medium-sized bowl. This should be enough for four small or two medium-sized salads.

## Breakfast Veggie Omelet

INGREDIENTS
Extra virgin olive oil spray
¼ to ½ cup cooked kale, spinach, chard, or broccoli rabe
2 eggs
Freshly ground black pepper
½ link chicken or turkey sausage, cut into 5 or 6 slices (optional)

Spray skillet (preferably nonstick) with a thin film of olive oil, then place over high heat. Warm cooked greens and/or sausage in a separate pan. Whisk together eggs with ground black pepper and pour mixture into hot skillet. As the eggs cook, carefully place the heated greens in a thick strip down the middle. Fold omelet around the greens and cook until done, about two to three minutes. Serve with sausages.

## Butternut Squash Soup

INGREDIENTS

Extra virgin olive oil spray

2 tsp. grated ginger

2 shallots, finely minced

3 12-ounce boxes of frozen winter squash

2½ cups soymilk

2½ cups chicken broth or vegetable broth

Salt to taste

In soup pan lightly sauté ginger and shallot in cooking spray. Thaw squash in microwave, purée, and add to pan. Continue to sauté for an additional three minutes. Add soymilk and broth to soup pan and stir. Bring to boil, add salt to taste, and serve. Serves 4.

## Flaxseed Toast

INGREDIENTS

1 cup flaxseed (preferably brown)

2 tbs. slivered almonds

½ tsp. garlic powder

½ tsp. lemon pepper

½ tsp. cumin seeds (optional)

Salt to taste

Roast flaxseed (1 minute in microwave on medium heat). Let seeds cool for 2 to 3 minutes. Grind the roasted flaxseed with the rest of the ingredients to a fine powder in a coffee grinder. This can be prepared the night before.

Serving Suggestion:

Add small amount of fat-free yogurt to the powder to use as a spread over 2 slices of toasted whole grain bread.

## Ginger and Garlic Greens

INGREDIENTS

4 9-ounce boxes of frozen spinach or broccoli (or 1lb. fresh)

3 tbs. extra virgin olive oil

2 tbs. grated ginger

2 tbs. minced garlic

Salt to taste

Combine above ingredients and heat in microwave ten minutes, stirring occasionally. Serves 4.

## Ginger-Garlic Salmon Fillets

INGREDIENTS

¼ cup extra virgin olive oil

1½ tsp. turmeric

1 tbs. minced garlic

1 tbs. grated ginger

1 tsp. cumin powder

Salt to taste

4 fillets of salmon (skin removed)

1 cup chicken or vegetable broth

Juice of 2 lemons

Combine oil, turmeric, garlic, ginger, cumin, and salt. Mix well. Spread mixture over salmon fillets, making sure to coat both sides. Marinate salmon one hour in refrigerator. Heat a large skillet over medium heat and place salmon fillets with marinade evenly spaced in skillet. Cook fillets four minutes on one side and three minutes on other side (heating time may vary). Remove fillets from pan. To make sauce, return pan to medium heat and whisk in broth, making sure to scrape up drippings from bottom of pan. Heat half a minute and pour sauce over salmon fillets. Sprinkle lemon juice over fillets. Serve over a bed of lettuce or brown rice. Serves 4.

## Greens Sautéed in Olive Oil and Garlic

INGREDIENTS

One bunch kale, chard (rainbow or Swiss), spinach, collards, mustard greens, or
    broccoli rabe
¼ cup extra virgin olive oil
2 cloves garlic, peeled and sliced about ¼ inch thick
Black pepper and salt to taste

You can use the same recipe for most greens, although some, like kale and collards, take longer to cook. You may choose to steam the greens before sautéing, but this recipe allows you to steam and sauté at the same time. Begin by rinsing greens in cold water and removing any black or brown patches. If kale or chard stems are thick or woody, peel leaves and tear into 2-inch pieces. In a nonstick covered casserole pan large enough to hold all the greens, pour olive oil over low heat and add sliced garlic. Simmer for several minutes until garlic begins to sizzle, but don't let it burn. Add greens still dripping and stir into the oil until they are well coated. Season with freshly ground black pepper and salt to taste. Cover pan and turn up the heat. The greens should have enough water from the rinsing to steam them, but you may need to keep a cup or two of water heating on the side and add before covering pan. Cook until the greens are wilted, checking occasionally for doneness. Serve immediately.

## Morning Tea

INGREDIENTS

½ cup water

1 green tea bag

½ cup soymilk

½ tsp. grated ginger

¼ tsp. sugar substitute, such as stevia

Bring water to a boil and pour over tea bag. Add soymilk, ginger, and sugar substitute.

## Spicy Mango and Strawberry Chutney

INGREDIENTS

4 ounces extra virgin olive oil

¼ tsp. turmeric

¼ tsp. red pepper flakes (optional)

2 tbs. fresh ginger, grated

Salt to taste

Pinch of sugar

12 ounces mango, cut into slices or cubes

4 ounces strawberries, cut into small pieces

Heat the oil in a microwave dish for thirty seconds. Add turmeric and red pepper flakes to the hot oil and mix. Add ginger, salt, sugar, and mango, then microwave for two minutes (until mango cubes are tender). Mash the mixture together into a thick paste. Fold in strawberries. Serves 4.

Serving Suggestions:
Serve with whole wheat pita crisps.
Put on takeout Tandoori chicken or made-at-home roast chicken.


## Tuna and Grape Tomatoes on Brown Rice

INGREDIENTS
1 cup extra virgin olive oil
2 tbs. minced garlic
3 6-ounce cans of tuna in water
2 cups grape tomatoes, cut in half
Salt to taste
2 cups cooked brown rice
⅓ cup fresh flat-leaf parsley, chopped (about 3 handfuls)
20 leaves of fresh basil, shredded

Heat a large, deep skillet over medium heat. Add oil and garlic to pan. When garlic starts sizzling in oil, add tuna and mash into oil with the back of a wooden spoon. Let the tuna sit in the oil five to ten minutes to infuse the fish flavor into the oil and to give the tuna time to break down; it will almost melt into the oil. Raise the flame a bit, and add the tomatoes to the pan. Season with salt. Heat the tomatoes through, about two minutes, and then add the cooked rice. Add parsley to the tuna and toss to combine well so that it evenly coats the rice. Adjust seasonings. Top rice with basil and serve. Serves 4.

# PART THREE

# THE ARTHRITIS
# Rx EXERCISES

# CHAPTER EIGHT

# EXERCISE SERIES A:
# RETURN TO MOVEMENT

When you are following the series of exercises laid out here, from Series A to Series C, remember to breathe deeply as you work out. If necessary, go back and reread the section on deep breathing in Chapter Three to refresh your memory. Naturally, you will not be able to breathe quite so deeply when you are doing stretches and exercises as when you are sitting in a chair. But the more you are able to breathe through the nose and down into the lower part of the lungs, the more you will benefit from doing these exercises.

## SUN SALUTATION LYING DOWN

The Sun Salutation Lying Down is a variation of the standing Sun Salutation with which yoga practitioners have been greeting the day for thousands of years. The most important modification is that the exercise is done flat on your back. The first half of the Series A routine is done in the same position to maximize support for, and minimize pressure on, the lower back and the lumbar vertebral disks.

- Lie flat on your back with your legs straight and your arms straight and long at your sides. Look up at the ceiling, so that your neck and back form one continuous line.

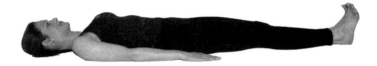

- Inhale as you sweep your arms out from your sides along the floor to point above your head. Imagine the line of your neck and spine becoming even longer and straighter.

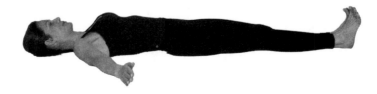

- Keeping your arms straight, sweep them up behind your head and slowly pull them back to your sides, with your palms flat on the floor. Exhale slowly and fully as you do this.

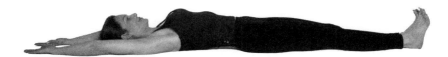

The Sun Salutation Lying Down is a warm-up stretch that prepares the body for action and sets the breathing tempo for all of Series A. If you like, you can do a series of Sun Salutations Lying Down until you feel your breathing settle into a slow, even tempo. Then you're ready to begin Series A in earnest.

## SINGLE LEG RAISE

- On the floor, lie flat with toes up. Bend your left knee and raise your right leg up straight with your toes flexed forward. Bring up to the level of your flexed knee and hold for five full breaths. Slowly bring your leg down.

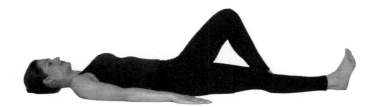

- Straighten your left leg. Bend your right knee and raise your left leg straight with your toes flexed forward. Bring up to the level of your flexed knee and hold for five full breaths. Slowly bring your leg down.

## ABDOMINAL CRUNCH

- Lie on the floor on your back with your arms at your sides and your palms flat on the floor. Slowly raise one knee and then the other to a bent position, with your feet flat on the floor.
- Inhale fully as you raise your shoulders off the floor and squeeze your abdominals. Don't raise your head first. Instead, try to keep your neck straight and let your head come up off the floor with your shoulders. If you lift your head high enough to bend your neck forward, not only will you work the abdominals less, but you will also slightly constrict your breathing and risk straining your neck muscles.

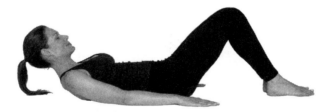

- Exhale slowly, then take four more full breaths, in and out, while you hold the stretch.
- Throughout the stretch, keep your palms, the insides of your forearms, and your elbows in contact with the floor. This focuses the exertion on isometrically contracting the oblique and upper abdominal muscles and on loosening the hip flexors.

- Relax back to the starting position as you take a sixth full breath.
- Straighten one leg and then the other from the bent-knee position.
- Perform another Sun Salutation Lying Down.

## KNEE TO CHEST

This exercise increases the stress on your abdominal muscles and begins to stretch them dynamically as well as isometrically.

- Lie on your back with your arms straight and long at your sides, your knees bent, and your feet flat on the floor. Point your toes straight ahead or turn them in slightly toward each other.
- Clasp your hands in the crook of one bent knee, and gently pull the knee toward your chest. Inhale slowly and fully as you reach the limit of your stretch, and raise your shoulders just off the floor to help open up the hip flexor. Point the toes of the raised foot toward the ceiling and try to hold your raised leg parallel to the floor, as if you were balancing a teacup on your shin.

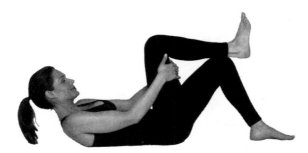

- Exhale slowly, and then hold the position at full stretch for four more deep breaths in and out.

- Relax back to the starting position as you take the sixth breath.
- Repeat the stretch with your other knee pulled to your chest.
- Perform a Sun Salutation Lying Down.

## ABDOMINAL CRUNCH WITH LEG FLEXED

- Lie flat on your back with your arms at your sides, palms on the floor. Gently raise one knee into a bent position while keeping your other leg straight, with the toes of the straight leg pointing to the ceiling.
- Inhale fully and gently, and raise your chest by bringing your shoulders off the floor. Keep your neck straight to facilitate breathing and try to raise your head and shoulders as one unit, or let your head lag slightly after your shoulders.

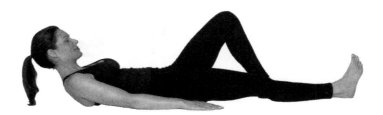

- Exhale slowly and hold the posture for four more breaths in and out.
- Relax back to the starting position, gently lowering your shoulders to the floor as your take a sixth breath.
- Repeat the stretch with your other knee bent.
- Perform another Sun Salutation Lying Down.

# TREE POSE

With the Tree Pose you're beginning to work the full hip musculature, including the hip flexors, abductors, external rotators, and extensors. In physical therapy, this is known as a classic FABERE (Flexion, Abduction, External Rotation, and Extension) stretch. The continuous breathing that Arthritis Rx adds to the stretch maximizes its benefit by driving more oxygen to the hip and pelvic areas.

- Lie flat on your back with your arms at your sides, palms facing down.
- As you inhale slowly and deeply, bend one leg and place the sole of that foot on the inside of your other knee. If you can't comfortably bring the sole of the foot as high as the knee, rest it against the inside of the lower leg.

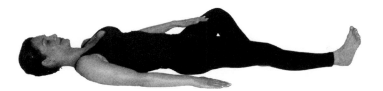

- Exhale slowly, and hold the position for four more breaths in and out.
- Look straight up at the ceiling and imagine your spine and neck lengthening in one continuous line.
- Relax back to the starting position as you take a sixth breath.
- Repeat the stretch with the other leg bent.
- Perform another Sun Salutation Lying Down.

## BOUND ANGLE POSTURE

The Bound Angle Posture is a FABERE stretch for both hips at once.

- Lie flat on your back with your arms at your sides, palms down.
- As you inhale slowly, draw one foot and then the other in toward your groin, so that your heels touch but your toes do not.

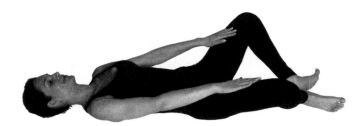

- Exhale slowly, and focus on the feeling of gravity pulling your knees to the floor. Imagine your knees spreading apart from each other like the opening of an Oriental fan. Keeping your heels together and making a V with your feet works in symbiosis with the knees to open up the hips.
- Hold the position for four more full breaths in and out.
- Relax to the starting position, slowly straightening your legs one at a time, as you take a sixth breath.
- Perform another Sun Salutation Lying Down.

## LUMBAR ROTATION DOUBLE KNEE

This posture works the abdominal obliques and begins to stretch the iliotibial band (ITB), which runs along the outside of your hip and thigh. The ITB is crucial to flexibility, and a tight ITB can cause sciatic symptoms. The Lumbar Rotation Double Knee also begins to stretch the paraspinal muscles, which run up and down both sides of the spine. As Arthritis Rx Series A continues, it gradually works more and more of the areas that are important for the body's flexibility, strength, and endurance.

- Lie on your back with your knees bent and feet flat on the floor, and extend your arms straight out from your shoulders.

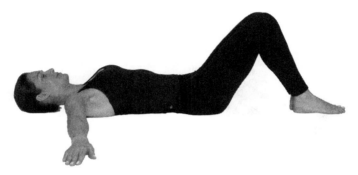

- Inhale fully and slowly lower your knees to one side, while keeping your shoulders flat to the floor. Don't force your knees down to the side. Let gravity do the work for you.

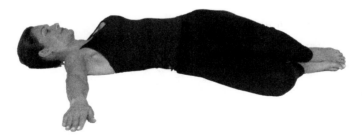

- Exhale, then hold the position for four more breaths in and out.
- Raise your knees back to the starting position as you take a sixth breath.
- Repeat the stretch by lowering your knees to the other side.
- Perform another Sun Salutation Lying Down.

# LUMBAR ROTATION SINGLE KNEE

This exercise increases the stretch of the ITB and the paraspinal muscles.

- After you finish the last Sun Salutation Lying Down, slowly turn onto one side and support your head on one hand. Place the other hand palm down in front of your chest and lean on it gently for support.

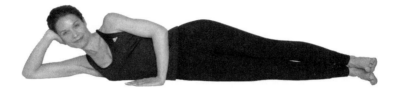

- Inhale fully, and cross your top leg over the bottom one so that your bent knee touches the floor in front of you at about waist level and your foot rests on the floor in front of the knee of your straight lower leg.

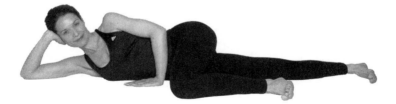

- Exhale, then hold the position for four more breaths in and out.
- Release the posture and turn gently onto your back as you take a sixth breath.
- Repeat on the other side.
- Perform another Sun Salutation Lying Down.

# HIP HIKERS

The Hip Hikers exercise helps to maximize the range of motion in your hips and is the most strenuous FABERE stretch in Series A. It concludes the supine warm-up period of the workout. The remaining exercises will be a little more heavy-duty.

- Take the same starting position as in the Lumbar Rotation Single Knee, lying on one side with one hand supporting your head and the other placed in front of your chest to support your whole body at a slight angle toward the floor.
- Keeping both legs straight, slowly raise one leg as you inhale fully.

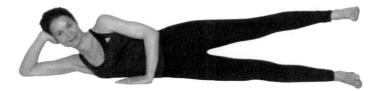

- Exhale, and hold the position for four more full breaths in and out, feeling the stretch in your hip and thigh.
- Gently lower the leg as you take a sixth breath.
- Repeat on your other side.
- Perform another Sun Salutation Lying Down.

## FINGERS TO TOES STRETCH

The Fingers to Toes Stretch stretches the hamstrings and calves of the legs.

- Sit with the toes pointed up, and slowly bend forward with both hands stretched out.

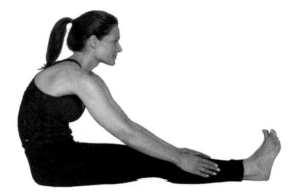

- Keep your spine straight and exhale.
- Hold for five full breaths and relax.
- Take a sixth breath.

## LOCUST POSTURE

This posture works both the paraspinal muscles and the abdominal muscles.

- Carefully move into a prone position, lying flat on the floor on your stomach with your arms straight and long at your sides.

- Keeping your knees straight, raise one leg off the floor as you inhale fully. You should feel the stretch in your hip. It does not matter how high you raise the leg, as long as you keep it straight and the knee is off the floor.

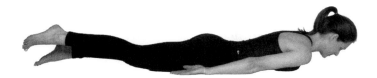

- Try to remain as relaxed as possible in the upper body and hold the position while taking four more full breaths in and out.
- Relax back to the starting position as you take a sixth breath.
- Repeat the exercise with the other leg.

## BACK EXTENSION

- Take a position on all fours, with your weight distributed evenly on your hands and knees.

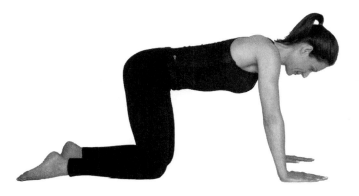

- Keeping your neck and back in line with each other, lift one leg and extend it backward as you inhale fully. Try to feel your neck and back lengthening into one continuous line with the extended leg. Don't cant or tip the hip of the extended leg out of a parallel line with the other hip, as that will put excessive strain on the canted side. Keeping the hips at the same level applies gentle, healing stress evenly across the whole back.

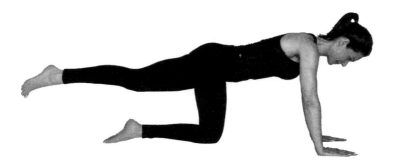

- Exhale slowly, then hold the position for four more breaths in and out.
- Relax back to the starting position on hands and knees as you take a sixth breath.
- Check to make sure your weight is once again distributed evenly on all fours, then repeat the posture by extending the other leg.

- Slowly stand up. Maintain straight posture. Slowly bring arms in front of you.

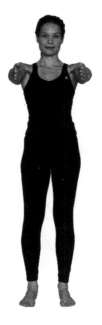

- Take left leg off ground and bend slowly.
- Slowly raise slightly bent left leg off the ground and hold for five deep breaths.

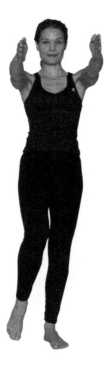

- Put left leg on ground and slowly lift right leg off the ground in slightly bent position and hold for five breaths.
- Now put both legs on the ground and take a breath.
- Perform a Sun Salutation Standing (see page 142).

# FLEXIBILITY PRAYER

The Flexibility Prayer introduces weight-bearing stretches of the paraspinal muscles, along with hip rotation and engagement of the oblique abdominal muscles.

- Stand up carefully with your feet the same width apart as your shoulder blades.
- Let your arms hang easily at your sides and try to make one continuous line of your spine and the back of your neck.
- Stretch your arms out in front of you with your palms together as if in prayer.
- Slowly turn your body as far as you can to one side as you inhale fully.
- Exhale, and hold the position for four more breaths in and out.
- Slowly turn to face front. Then turn to the other side, and hold the position for five more deep breaths in and out.
- Relax back to the starting position with your arms at your sides.

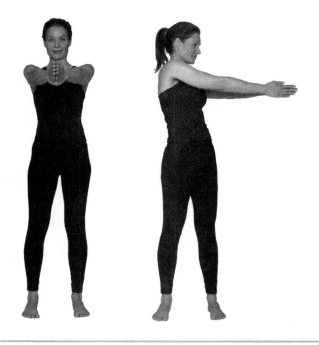

# SUN SALUTATION STANDING

- Take the same starting position as in the Flexibility Prayer, standing straight and tall with your feet about the same width apart as your shoulder blades.
- Sweep your arms up to your sides and above your head as you inhale fully.
- Sweep your straight arms down in front of you to return to rest at your sides as you exhale slowly.

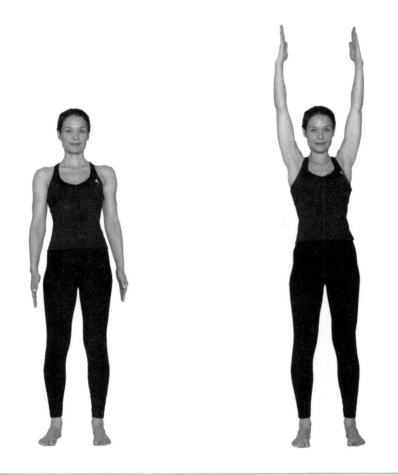

## STANDING TREE POSE

This difficult posture fires all the core muscle groups in proper sequence. Don't try to hold the posture for five full breaths when you first do it. Start with three breaths and work your way up.

- Stand straight and tall with your feet about the same width apart as your shoulder blades. Keep your neck straight so that you are looking directly in front of you, as if at the distant horizon.

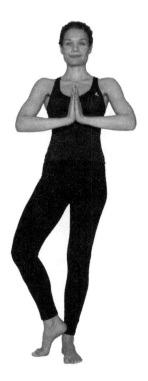

- Bring the heel of one foot up to rest on the ankle of the other leg, with the ball of the foot continuing to touch the floor.

- Inhale slowly as you raise your arms to reach for the sky.

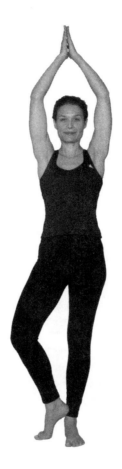

- Exhale slowly, and take two more deep breaths in and out.
- Relax to the starting position as you take a fourth full breath.
- Repeat with the other heel raised to rest on your other ankle.
- Perform a Sun Salutation Standing.

Congratulations! You've now completed Arthritis Rx Series A.

# CHAPTER NINE

# EXERCISE SERIES B:
# RESUMING FULL ACTIVITY

---

Arthritis Rx Series B will help you complete your recovery and return to an active lifestyle. The Series B exercises build on the Series A exercises in two ways: The postures themselves are a little more difficult, and the routine calls for holding every posture for seven full breaths instead of five.

# SUN SALUTATION LYING DOWN

- Lie flat on your back with your legs straight and your arms straight and long at your sides. Look straight up at the ceiling so that your neck and back form one continuous line.

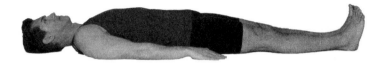

- Sweep your arms out from your sides along the floor to point straight back above your head. Inhale as you do, so that the lungs fill completely as your arms point straight back behind you. Imagine the straight line of your neck and spine becoming even longer and straighter.

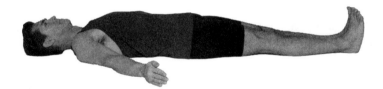

- Keeping your arms straight, sweep them up behind your head, raise them up toward the ceiling, and slowly let gravity carry them back to your sides, with your palms flat on the floor. Exhale slowly and fully as you do this.

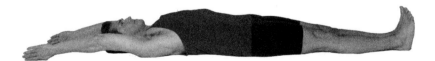

# SINGLE LEG RAISE

- Lie on the floor. Bend your left knee and raise your right leg up to the level of your left knee.

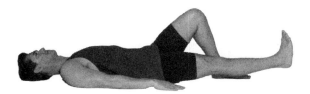

- Take a deep breath. As you exhale, lower your right leg toward the ground, but don't touch it.

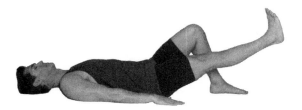

- As you inhale, raise your right leg up to the level of your left knee.
- Perform four more times and repeat on other side. You will do seven repetitions on each side.

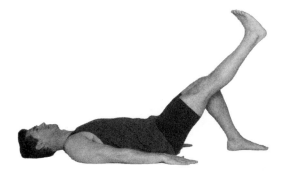

# INTERMEDIATE ABDOMINAL CRUNCH

In this posture and the ones immediately following, crossing your arms on your chest, instead of resting them on the floor at your sides, will isolate the abdominal muscles and work them harder than the corresponding Series A postures.

- Lie on the floor on your back with your arms crossed on your chest, and then slowly raise one knee and then the other to a bent position, with your feet flat on the floor.
- Inhale fully as you raise your shoulders off the floor and squeeze your abdominals. Don't raise your head first. Instead, try to keep your neck straight and let your head and shoulders come up off the floor as a unit.
- Exhale slowly, then take six more full breaths in and out while you hold the stretch.
- Relax back to the starting position as you take an eighth full breath.
- Straighten one leg and then the other from the bent knee position.
- Perform another Sun Salutation Lying Down.

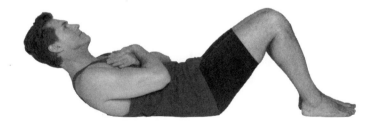

# KNEE TO CHEST WITH FEET FLEXED

- Lie flat on your back with your arms crossed over your chest and your legs straight. Flex your feet so that your toes point straight to the ceiling.
- Lift one knee and bring it as close to your chest as possible. Inhale slowly and fully as you press to the limit of your stretch, and raise your shoulders just off the floor to help open up the hip flexor. Point the toes of the raised foot toward the ceiling and try to hold your raised leg parallel to the floor, as if you were balancing a teacup on your shin.

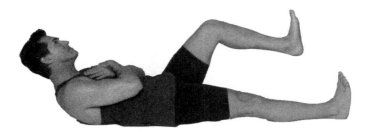

- Exhale slowly, then hold the position at full stretch for six more deep breaths in and out.
- Relax back to the starting position as you take your eighth breath.
- Repeat the stretch with your other knee pulled to your chest.
- Perform a Sun Salutation Lying Down.

## INTERMEDIATE ABDOMINAL CRUNCH WITH LEG FLEXED

- Lie flat on your back with your arms crossed on your chest. Gently raise one knee into a bent position. Lift your other leg, keeping it flexed straight, until your thighs are parallel with each other.

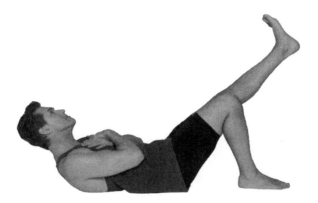

- Inhale fully and gently raise your chest by bringing your shoulders off the floor. Keep your neck straight to facilitate breathing, and try to raise your head and shoulders as one unit, or let your head lag slightly after your shoulders.
- Exhale slowly, and hold the posture for six more full breaths in and out.
- Relax back to the starting position, gently lowering your shoulders to the floor as you take an eighth breath.
- Repeat the stretch with your other knee bent.
- Perform a Sun Salutation Lying Down.

## TREE POSE WITH LEG CROSSED

- Lie flat on your back with your arms at your sides, palms facing down.
- As you inhale slowly and deeply, bend one leg and rest that foot on the top of your other knee. This opens up the hip flexor and lets gravity give you more of a stretch than in the Series A Tree Pose.

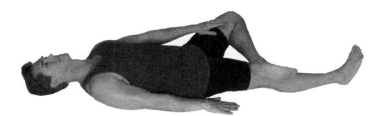

- Exhale slowly, and hold the position for six more full breaths in and out.
- Look straight up at the ceiling and imagine your spine and neck lengthening in one continuous line.
- Relax back to the starting position as you take an eighth breath.
- Repeat the stretch with the other leg bent.
- Perform a Sun Salutation Lying Down.

## BOUND ANGLE POSTURE WITH FEET TOGETHER

- Lie flat on your back with your arms at your sides, palms down.
- As you inhale slowly, draw one foot at a time in toward your groin so that the soles of your feet touch. Imagine that the soles of your feet are glued together; this opens up the hip flexors more than the Series A Bound Angle Posture, where the feet form a V.

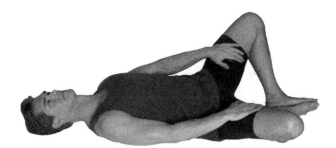

- Exhale slowly, and focus on the feeling of gravity pulling your knees to the floor. Imagine your knees spreading apart from each other like the opening of an Oriental fan.
- Hold the position for six more full breaths in and out.
- Relax to the starting position, slowly straightening your legs one at a time, as you take an eighth breath.
- Perform another Sun Salutation Lying Down.

## LUMBAR ROTATION WITH LEG CROSSED

- Lie flat on your back with your legs straight and your arms extended straight out to the sides.
- Slowly raise one leg into a bent knee position with your foot flat on the floor on the outside of your other knee.
- Inhale fully, and let gravity pull your bent knee down to the floor to the outside of the straight leg.

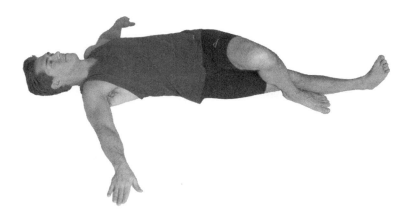

- Exhale slowly, then hold the position for six more deep breaths in and out.
- Relax back to the starting position as you take an eighth breath.
- Repeat with the other knee raised.
- Perform another Sun Salutation Lying Down.

## SIDE TREE

- Lie on your side with your head supported by one hand and the other palm flat on the floor in front of your chest, supporting your body.
- Inhale fully as your raise your upper leg into a bent knee position and rest the sole of that foot on the floor in front of your straight knee.

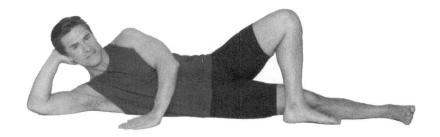

- Exhale slowly, and hold the position for six more deep breaths in and out.
- Relax back to the starting position as you take an eighth breath.
- Carefully turn over onto your other side and repeat the posture with your opposite leg.
- Perform another Sun Salutation Lying Down.

## INTERMEDIATE HIP HIKES

- Lie on your right side with one hand supporting your head and the other placed in front of your chest to support your whole body at a slight angle toward the floor.

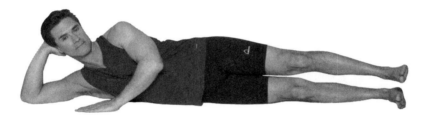

- Keep both legs straight, and slowly raise your left leg as you inhale fully.
- Exhale, and hold the position for six more full breaths in and out, feeling the stretch in your hip and thigh.

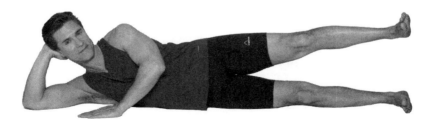

- Gently lower your leg as you take an eighth breath.
- Repeat seven times. Don't touch your right foot as you lower your left leg.
- Carefully turn over onto your left side, and repeat the exercise with the right leg seven times.
- Perform another Sun Salutation Lying Down.

## FINGERS TO TOES

- Sit with your toes pointed up, and slightly bend forward with both hands stretched out.
- Try to touch your toes.
- Repeat seven times.

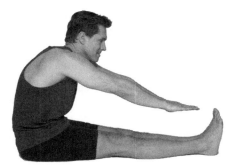

## INTERMEDIATE LOCUST POSTURE

- Carefully move into a prone position, lying flat on the floor on your stomach with your legs straight and arms fully extended.
- Keeping your knees straight, raise one leg and the opposite arm off the floor as you inhale fully. It does not matter how high you raise the leg and opposite arm, as long as you keep them straight and both the knee and elbow are off the floor. Raising the opposite arm and leg together stretches the abdominal wall more fully than the Series A posture. It also engages the whole back rather than focusing solely on the lower back.

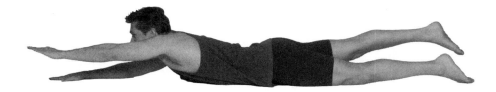

- Exhale slowly, and hold the position for six more full breaths in and out.
- Relax back to the starting position as you take an eighth breath.
- Repeat the exercise with the other leg.


## INTERMEDIATE BACK EXTENSION

- Take a position on all fours, with your weight distributed evenly on your hands and knees.
- Keep your neck and back in line with each other. Inhale fully as you lift one leg and extend it backward, and raise the opposite arm and reach forward. Try to feel your neck and back lengthening into one continuous line with the extended

leg. Don't cant or tip the hip of the extended leg out of a parallel line with the other hip, as that will put excessive strain on the canted side.

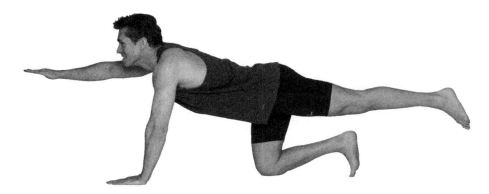

- Exhale slowly, then hold the position for six more breaths in and out.
- Relax back to the starting position on hands and knees as you take an eighth breath.
- Check to make sure your weight is once again distributed evenly on all fours. Then repeat the posture by extending the other leg and arm.

# SINGLE LEG STAND

- Slowly stand up. Maintain straight posture. Slowly bring arms out in front of you.

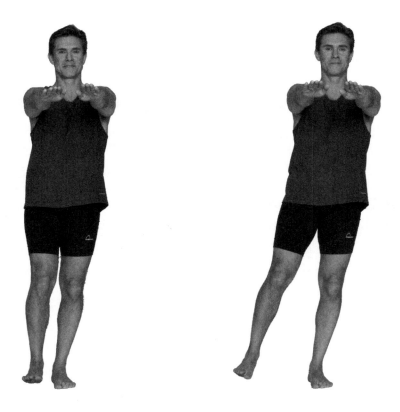

- Slowly raise slightly bent left leg off the ground and hold for seven deep breaths.
- Put left leg on ground and slowly lift right leg off the ground in slightly bent position and hold for seven breaths.
- Now put both legs on the ground and take a breath.
- Repeat seven times.
- Perform a Sun Salutation Standing (see p. 159).

# SUN SALUTATION STANDING

- Stand straight and tall with your feet together or about the same width apart as your shoulder blades, whichever is more comfortable.
- Sweep your arms up to the sides and above your head as you inhale fully.
- Sweep your straight arms down in front of you to return to rest at your sides as you exhale slowly.

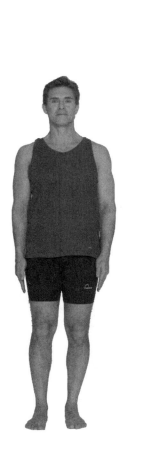 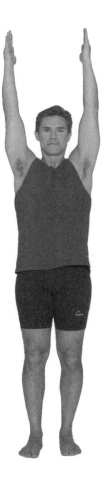

# STANDING TWIST

- Stand straight and tall with your feet about the same width apart as your shoulder blades, and rest your hands on your hips. Compared to the Flexibility Prayer in Series A, this limits your shoulder turn and increases your spinal twist.
- Rotate as far as possible to one side as you inhale fully.
- Exhale slowly, then hold the position for six more deep breaths in and out.
- Relax back to the starting position as you take an eighth breath.
- Rotate to the other side, holding the position for seven full breaths in and out.
- Perform a Sun Salutation Standing.

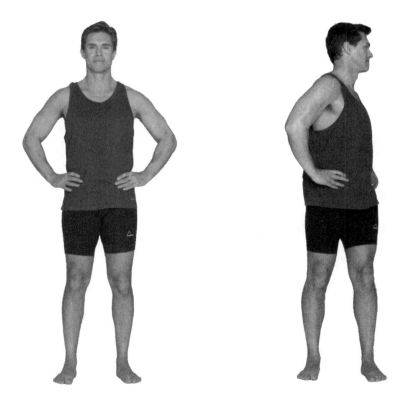

# STANDING TREE POSE

- Stand straight and tall with your feet about the same width apart as your shoulder blades. Keep your neck straight so that you are looking directly in front of you, as if at the distant horizon.
- Bring the sole of one foot up to rest against the knee of the other leg.
- Inhale slowly as you raise your arms to reach for the sky.

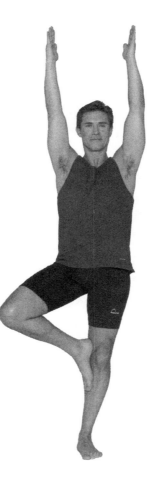

- Exhale slowly, and take six more deep breaths in and out. To maximize your proprioception, try to do this with your eyes closed.
- Relax to the starting position as you take an eighth full breath.
- Repeat with the other leg.
- Perform a Sun Salutation Standing.

You've now completed Arthritis Rx Series B. Doing this workout consistently every day, assuming you can first do Series A totally pain-free, should bring you back to full freedom of movement and enable you to resume all your normal activities, including recreational sports, usually in about two to four weeks.

# CHAPTER TEN

# EXERCISE SERIES C:
# INTO THE FAST LANE

This demanding routine should be started only if you can do Arthritis Rx Series B totally pain-free. It is done without Sun Salutations to set and reset a good breathing tempo, so it really works your proprioception and mind-body focus as well as your flexibility, strength, and endurance. If you are ready, it is an enormously rewarding challenge.

Series C requires you to hold each position or to continue each movement (the greater Pilates component in Series C means much more dynamic muscle work than in Series A or B) for ten deep, full breaths in and out. This is a goal to work toward, not something you have to achieve on the first try. More difficult than holding each position or continuing each movement for ten full breaths is keeping a steady breathing flow throughout the whole routine. As you get comfortable with the routine, strive to move more and more smoothly and continuously from one exercise to another, without having to pause to catch your breath or rest. Series C will really build your lung capacity, which is highly important to overall health.

The whole routine should take about fifteen to twenty minutes. Once again, however, while you are doing the exercises, watch your breathing, not the clock.

## THE HUNDRED

- Lie flat on your back with your knees bent, feet flat on the floor.
- Reach your hands toward your knees. The reach is from the shoulder, and your shoulders should come off the floor before your head does.
- Maintaining that extended reach from the shoulder, beat both arms down and up parallel to each other, keeping a strong, steady rhythm for ten full breaths in and out.
- Relax flat on your back as you take an eleventh breath.

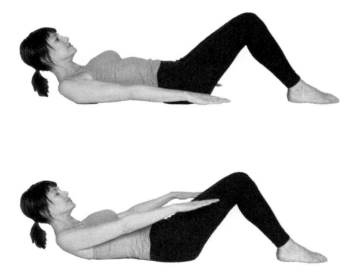

# ADVANCED CRUNCH

- Lie flat on your back with your knees bent and your arms crossed over your chest.
- Bring your shoulders off the floor and gently twist one shoulder toward the opposite knee. Hold the twist for ten full breaths. This really works the internal and external obliques.
- Relax back to the starting position as you take an eleventh breath. Then bring your shoulders off the floor again and repeat the twist on the other side. Hold this counter-twist for ten full breaths (if you cannot hold the position for a full ten breaths at first, make sure to keep the number of breaths on each side consistent).
- Relax back to the starting position as you take an eleventh breath.

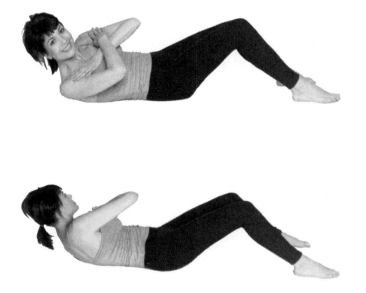

# CRISS-CROSS

- Lie flat on your back with your knees bent and your hands clasped under your head. The center of your lower back should remain flat on the floor for the entire exercise, as if it were glued to the floor.
- Straighten one leg, and point your toes to two o'clock, keeping your thighs parallel with each other. Pointing the toes throughout the exercise will develop a greater range of motion in the hip.
- Now get a bicycling motion going with your legs. Straighten each leg in turn as if you were trying to touch the two o'clock position with the tips of your toes. At the farthest stretch you want to have a straight line from the top of your big toe to the top of the thigh. Imagine beads of water dropping on your toe and running smoothly down that line in single file, without a single bump to interrupt or divert them.
- Keeping your shoulders straight, bring your upper body into play by alternately twisting up on each side and reaching your elbow toward your opposite knee. You should eventually be able to touch your knee with the tip of your elbow. Don't let your elbows fold in toward each other as you do this exercise; it is important to keep them fanned out as much as possible. Your elbows should stay even with your ears so that your upper arms form a single straight line with your shoulders.
- Continue the alternating movement for ten deep, rhythmic breaths.

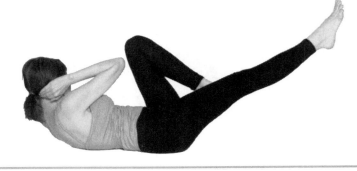

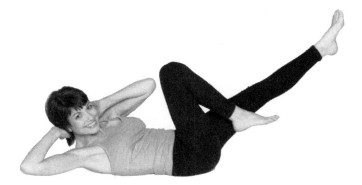

## REVERSE CRUNCH

- Lie flat on your back with your arms straight and long at your sides, palms flat on the floor.
- Curl your knees up toward your chest as if you were going to roll into a reverse somersault. As your knees roll up over your chest, straighten your legs and try to touch the ceiling with the balls of your feet.

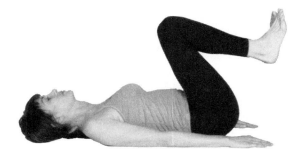

- Take ten full breaths in and out, and keep reaching for the ceiling with the balls of your feet. Your knees should remain in line with your chest.
- Relax back into a bent knee position with your feet flat on the floor as you take an eleventh breath.

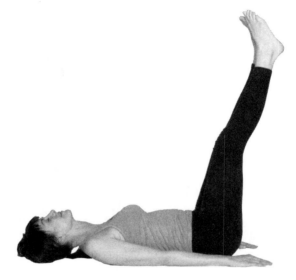

## CIRCLES

- Lie flat on your back with your arms straight and long at your sides, palms flat on the floor. Stretch your legs out as long as possible, flex your feet forward, and point your toes straight ahead. Then raise one leg into a bent knee position with your foot flat on the floor.
- Swing the bent leg up into the air and take it through as wide a circular arc as you can. Flex the foot and point your toes. This stretches the hip flexors to their

maximum, developing an increased range of motion in the hip. The movement also gives a good workout to your lower abdominals and obliques.

- Continue circling the leg around for ten full breaths in and out.
- Relax back to the starting position.
- Repeat the exercise with your other leg for ten full breaths in and out.

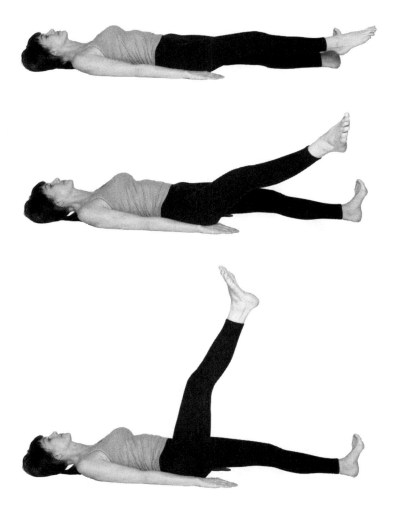

## HAMSTRING STRETCH LYING DOWN

- Lie flat on your back with your arms straight and long at your sides, palms flat on the floor. Raise your knees into a bent position with your feet flat on the floor.
- Lift one leg, clasp your hands behind your knee, and pull gently.
- In this exercise, don't point your toes to the ceiling. Instead, keep the sole of your foot parallel to the floor, as if you were trying to balance a teacup on your toes. Your shoulders should stay flat to the floor, as if they were glued there, and the opposite foot should also be grounded firmly but gently, sole flat on the floor.
- Hold the stretch for ten deep breaths in and out.
- Repeat with your other leg for ten deep breaths in and out.

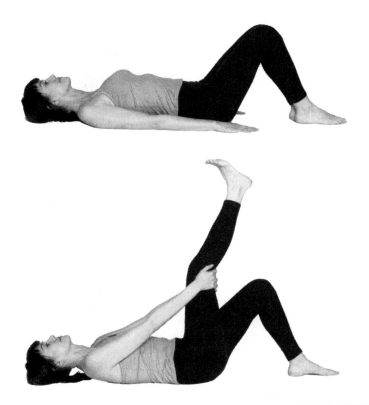

# ADVANCED BRIDGING

- Lie flat on your back with your arms straight and long at your sides, palms flat on the floor, and raise your knees into a bent position.
- Straighten one leg and point your toes, keeping your thighs parallel to each other.
- Tighten your buttocks, pull in your abdominal muscles, and roll your hips upward until your pelvis forms a straight line with your thighs.
- Repeat with the other leg straightened out.

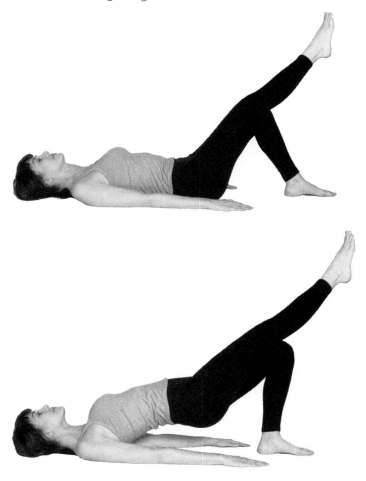

## HAMSTRING STRETCH SEATED

- Sit down on the floor with your legs extended straight in front of you, toes pointed to the ceiling. Rest your palms flat on the floor beside your knees.
- Bend one leg and place the sole of that foot against the inside of your other knee. The side of the bent knee should touch the floor if possible.
- Keeping your back straight, lean forward as far as possible from the waist. As you lean forward, your chest and abdominals should lead the way, and your head, neck, and shoulders should follow. Try to keep your arms straight, too, sliding your palms forward a little as you lean into the stretch.

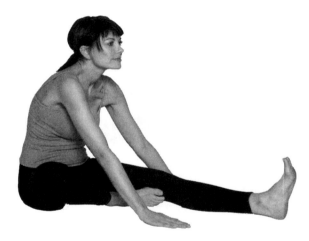

## UPWARD-FACING DOG

- Lie flat on your stomach with your toes pointed straight back and your hands tucked under your shoulders.
- Feel your back and your neck forming one long line, and raise your upper body in one unit from the waist.
- Don't push up with your arms. But let them straighten and support you gently as you feel the stretch in the small of your back and your hips. Your neck should form a single line with your back, and your gaze should be straight ahead, as if looking at the distant horizon. This keeps your neck relaxed and open to facilitate good breathing.
- Hold the position at the limit of your stretch for ten full breaths in and out.

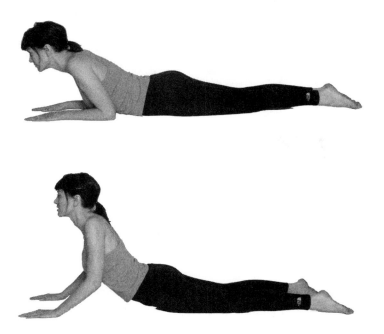

## PRONE LEG BEATS

- Lie flat on your stomach with your toes pointing straight back and your hands folded underneath your chin. Your heels should be touching.
- Raise both legs off the ground, keeping them together and straight.
- As you take ten full breaths in and out, tap your heels together.

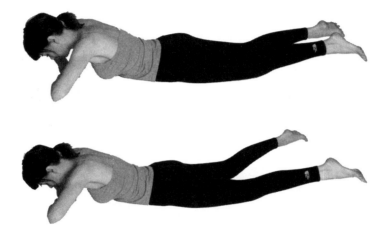

## ALTERNATING SUPERMAN

- Lie on your stomach straight and long, with your toes pointed behind you and your arms extended in front of you, palms flat on the floor.
- Scissor your arms and legs at a steady, rhythmic beat for ten full breaths in and out.

- You shouldn't feel any strain in your neck. Try to keep your neck open and relaxed so that it seems to form a continuous line with your spine.

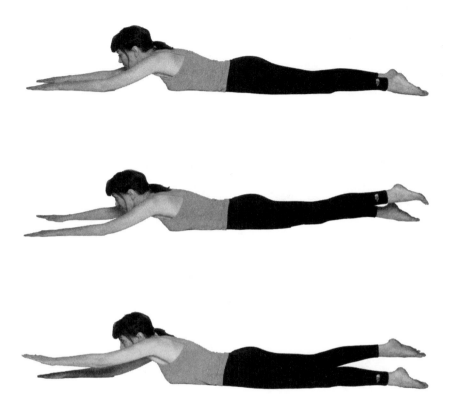

# KNEE TO CHEST ON ALL FOURS

- Take a position on all fours, with your weight evenly distributed on your hands and knees.
- Arch your back into a gentle C-shape, and pull one knee toward your chest.
- Hold the knee as close to your chest as possible for ten full breaths in and out.
- Repeat with your other leg for ten full breaths in and out.

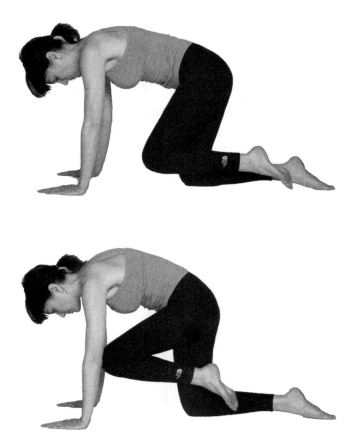

## FIERCE (UNEVEN) POSTURE

- Stand up straight and tall, with your feet about the same width apart as your shoulder blades, and reach up as if you were trying to touch the ceiling with the tips of your fingers. Pigeon-toe your feet slightly, or point them straight ahead.
- Keeping your back and neck as straight as possible, sit down as if there were a chair right under you. Pretend that the seat of the chair is dropping ever so slowly to the floor, and try to catch up with it so that it can support your weight.
- This is a very simple-looking posture. But the fitter you are, the more you can benefit from it.

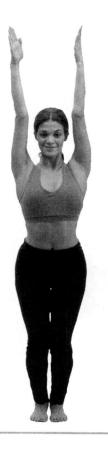

# ADVANCED STANDING TREE POSE

- Stand straight and tall with your feet about the same width apart as your shoulder blades. Keep your neck straight, as if you were gazing at the distant horizon.
- Bring the sole of one foot up to rest against the knee of the other leg.
- Inhale slowly as you raise your arms to reach for the sky.
- Bring your palms together above your head.
- Exhale slowly, and take nine more deep breaths in and out. To maximize your proprioception, try to do this with your eyes closed.
- Relax to the starting position as you take an eleventh full breath.
- Repeat with the other leg.

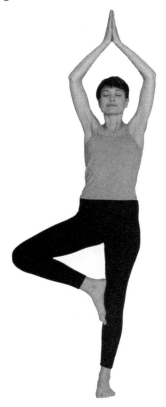

# CHAPTER ELEVEN

# TREATING WRIST, HAND, FOOT, ANKLE, NECK, AND SHOULDER ARTHRITIS

Arthritis is an equal opportunity destroyer. Not content to attack the knees of 18 million Americans, the lower backs of 16 million, and the hips of 15 million, it has delivered pain and immobility to many millions more through the other joints of the body. Arthritis of the shoulder afflicts about 2½ million Americans; neck arthritis, nearly 3 million; arthritis of the foot and ankle claims another 5 million; and wrist-hand arthritis as many as 10 million (according to the National Institutes of Health). Arthritis may affect any joint in the body. It most often occurs in the weight-bearing joints, the hip and knee. But it may also strike other joints in the hands, shoulders, and feet. The hands are prime targets for the non-weight-bearing joints of the upper limbs.

The Framingham Study found that 26 percent of women and 13 percent of men over age seventy had arthritis in at least one finger joint. Arthritis robs hands of strength, making it difficult to grip pens, open jars, and turn keys. The condition most often develops at the base of the thumb, at the middle of a finger, and at the fingertip. The dominant hand is most likely to be affected. In addition to the stretch shown at the end of this chapter, one of the best exercises for hand arthritis is to get a sponge and submerge your hand and wrist completely in warm water. In the water you should squeeze the sponge ten times slowly, rest a moment, then repeat this at least five times. This simple exercise will help maintain strength of the arthritic hand while minimizing symptoms. The Arthritis Rx supplement also has tremendous benefit for hand arthritis as it helps to keep the inflammation down in the arthritic joint, resulting in less pain and better motion. I have found acupuncture to be of great benefit to patients suffering from hand and wrist arthritis, when combined with the exercises and supplements in my plan.

Like other forms of arthritis, hand arthritis often appears after years of typing, playing stringed instruments, or engaging in other activities that have irritated and worn away the cartilage in the fingers and wrists. Being double-jointed, however, may offer some protection. According to a recent study in *Arthritis & Rheumatism*, forty- to ninety-year-olds who were double-jointed were less likely to develop arthritis of the PIP (proximal interphalangeal) joint in the middle of the finger. This was good news: The PIP joint plays a key role in the ability to grip and pinch. New studies are underway, including one at our institution, to evaluate the role of joint lubricants such as hylan in treating arthritis of the hand, with some promising early results. In addition, you may want to seek out so-called adaptive clothing specially designed for people with limited use of their hands from companies such as Pep-Ease (pepease.com).

Like hand arthritis, shoulder arthritis may interfere with the ability to perform common activities such as combing one's hair or reaching for an object. The shoulder consists of the largest and most movable joints in the body. Although most people assume it is a single joint, it consists of two: the acromioclavicular, or AC, joint, which is located where the collarbone (clavicle) meets the tip of the shoulder bone (acromion); and the glenohumeral joint, which is located at the junction of the upper arm bone (humerus) with the shoulder blade (scapula). The glenohumeral joint helps move the shoulder forward and backward and allows the arm to rotate in a circular fashion or hinge out and up and away from the body.

Arthritis is more common in the AC joint than in the glenohumeral joint. Individuals who have suffered a fracture or dislocation of the shoulder often develop arthritis of the shoulder later in life. Arthritis can also develop in the shoulder after a tear in the rotator cuff tendon.

If the glenohumeral joint is affected, pain occurs in the back of the shoulder. If the AC joint is the problem, pain is concentrated in the front of the shoulder. The pain often intensifies after simple activities, and is often intense enough to interrupt sleep. Some people hear a clicking sound when they move. I have had excellent results by combining massage therapy with physical therapy in the treatment of shoulder arthritis. A multi-center trial is currently underway, sponsored by Sanofi Corp., to evaluate the role of the joint lubricant hylan in treating shoulder arthritis. We have done this procedure on fifty patients with shoulder arthritis here with very promising early results. If there is no relief from such intervention, total shoulder replacement should be considered.

Neck arthritis is another frequent cause of chronic pain among adults. Bony spurs, injuries to the ligaments, and diseases can lead to chronic pain and stiffness in the neck. Some people with neck arthritis find that the pain intensifies when they engage in activities such as working at a computer, which requires the same upright position for long periods. Muscle spasms are common in neck arthritis, and many people with arthritic necks hear popping sounds when they change position. Acupuncture and physical therapy that utilizes traction have yielded good results among patients I have worked with.

By age sixty, half of the population has arthritis in one of the thirty-three joints of the foot. Being overweight increases the risk, as extra pounds contribute to the deterioration of cartilage and the development of bone spurs. A severe injury or a history of previous injuries from playing sports may make the foot vulnerable to arthritis. Arthritis of the foot contributes to the loss of mobility, making it difficult to walk even short distances. Foot pain often causes people to change the way they turn their ankles, knees, and hips. As a result, these joints are under stress, which can contribute to the deterioration of the cartilage in these joints as well. One of the best exercises for foot and ankle arthritis is to submerge the limb in lukewarm water (make sure to check the water temperature with the hands first) up to the calf and draw the alphabet with your toes at the bottom of the bucket or tub, one letter at a time. This will maintain the flexibility and strength of the arthritic foot or ankle joint.

Orthotic devices may be used to help individuals cope with arthritis of the feet. These devices range from footpads or heel inserts purchased at local pharmacies to custom-molded, individually designed shoe inserts or ankle braces provided by a podiatrist, a professional who has had extensive training and experience in managing foot and ankle problems. The type of device recommended by your physician will depend on your symptoms, the shape of your feet, and other factors. Custom-made orthotic devices provide more support and correction than off-the-shelf devices do. In the past, plaster molds of the foot were used to construct the custom-made devices, but now computerized foot analysis is often employed to develop devices that closely reflect the dynamics of the patient's gait.

Dr. Rock G. Positano, my colleague at the Hospital for Special Surgery and director of the Non-operative Foot and Ankle Service at New York Presbyterian Hospital/Weill-Cornell Medical Center, cautions, "Orthotics are definitely a prescription item that requires expert diagnosis and fitting. Inserts that you buy over-the-counter or over the Internet can easily worsen the problem you are trying to correct."

I have found that combining the use of orthotics with the application of heat in the morning and ice at night is helpful in treating symptoms of ankle and toe arthritis. Ultrasound therapy, a modality that uses sound waves to create deep heat in the affected tissues, is a useful adjunct to orthotic treatments. My colleagues at HSS and I have had successful early results in treating foot and ankle arthritis with hylan injections when combined with the Arthritis Rx Plan. We are in the process of setting up a trial on the role of hylan in ankle arthritis with the Genzyme Corporation. Surgery usually means fusing the painful ankle or toe joint, and is the last option for treating foot and ankle arthritis. All non-surgical conservative measures should be tried first.

Indeed, to relieve the pain of foot, hand, shoulder, and neck joints, we always begin with more conservative measures. The Arthritis Rx Plan can help these joints as well as those of the hip and knee. Exercise helps maintain joint flexibility and conditions the muscles that support the arthritic joint. Hot and cold packs enable many individuals with these joint problems to reduce pain and inflammation. Some individuals also use NSAIDs, or the prescription COX-2 inhibitors, which offer pain relief similar to that of NSAIDs but without the gastrointestinal side effects. Corticosteroids are used for a small percentage of arthritis patients; those who have acute flare-ups or those who have significant swelling in the joint.

As I noted earlier in my discussion of treating hip and knee arthritis, hyaluronic acid (HA) is a normal component of the joint involved in joint lubrication. Injections of synthetic HA, called hylan, are now being tried increasingly for arthritis of the shoulder, foot and ankle, and wrist and hand. Patients receive three to five injections over several weeks. They may have to avoid heavy lifting or other physically demanding activities for the first forty-eight hours after the injection, but effects may last for several months. The injections don't reverse arthritis, although early evidence indicates that they may delay its progression. Side effects are rare; the most common one is swelling at the injection site. Early experiences at our institution for treating shoulder, hand, and foot and ankle arthritis have been promising. At HSS, we have treated about eighty shoulders, fifty ankles, twenty-five toes, and twenty hands, with the majority of patients reporting excellent results. The multi-center trial sponsored by Sanofi Corp. involving major medical institutions using hylan in the shoulder has had similarly positive results. In the future, I expect hylan therapy to be used more frequently for arthritis of these joints as more data is gathered on its usefulness.

Another new therapy that is being used for arthritis in the spine that has not responded to conservative therapies is radio frequency denervation. Using X-ray guidance, the physician places a needle in a catheter at the site of the nerve that is transmitting joint pain. Heat is used to deaden the nerve. The treatment lasts up to twenty-four months. Our studies published in the journal *Pain Physician* in 2003 showed an 80 percent success rate with this technology. (For more information on radio frequency denervation, refer to my first book, *Back Rx* [Gotham Books, 2004].) If there is no relief with radio frequency denervation, fusing of the spine is the only option left to alleviate pain. The success rate for spine fusion for neck pain alone remains around 50 percent. Combining different integrative therapies with the Arthritis Rx Plan will give pain relief to the vast majority of those afflicted with arthritis of the wrist and hand, neck and shoulder, foot and toes, and will lead to decreased pain, enhanced mobility, and the slowing of the progression of the disease.

Now let's look at simple stretches to maintain the strength and flexibility of the arthritic wrist and hand, the arthritic neck, the arthritic shoulder, and finally the arthritic foot and ankle.

# RESOURCES FOR FURTHER INFORMATION AND TREATMENT OF ARTHRITIS OF THE OTHER JOINTS:

## *Wrist and hand*

American Society for Surgery of the Hand     assh.org

## *Foot and ankle*

American Podiatric Medical Association     apma.org
American Orthopaedic Foot & Ankle Society     aofas.org

## *Shoulder*

American Shoulder and Elbow Surgeons     ases-assn.org

## *Neck*

American Academy of Physical Medicine and
    Rehabilitation     aapmr.org
Physiatric Association of Spine, Sports and
    Occupational Rehabilitation     aapmr.org/passor.htm
North American Spine Society     spine.org

## WRIST STRETCH

- Hold your left arm straight out in front of you, palm up. Using your right hand, gently pull down on the fingers of the left hand as much as you can until your fingers point toward the floor.
- Hold for twenty seconds.
- Repeat three times.
- Repeat exercise on other hand.

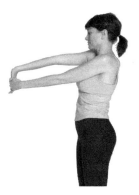

## HAND EXERCISE

This simple exercise will help maintain the strength of the arthritic hand while minimizing symptoms.

- Grasp a sponge with your affected hand and submerge your hand and wrist completely in warm water.
- Under the water, squeeze the sponge ten times slowly, then rest a moment.
- Repeat this at least five times.

# NECK STRETCH

- Start with the head erect and chin jutting as far forward as is comfortable.
- Pull chin back toward the neck so that it points to the supersternal notch at the top of the breastbone, but does not touch it.
- Hold for twenty seconds.
- Repeat three times.

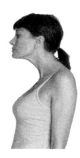 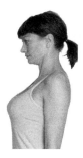

## SHOULDER STRETCH LYING DOWN

- Lie flat on your back.
- Reach your left arm across your chest so that the palm touches the floor beyond your right shoulder.
- Place your right hand on your left elbow and push your elbow down into your chest.
- Hold for twenty seconds.
- Repeat three times.
- Repeat exercise on the other side.

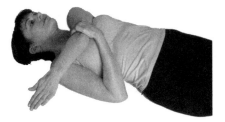

## FOOT AND ANKLE EXERCISE

- Submerge the limb in lukewarm water up to the calf in a bathtub or large basin.
- Draw each letter of the alphabet with your toes at the bottom of the basin or tub, one letter at a time.

# PART FOUR

# THE OTHER STAGES OF JOINT PAIN CARE AND RECOVERY

# CHAPTER TWELVE

# STAGE TWO CARE:
# ORAL MEDICATIONS
# AND INTEGRATIVE CARE

Clearly I believe that the full implementation of the Arthritis Rx Plan represents the best option for most arthritis sufferers. It is especially effective if you begin to follow the diet, supplement, and exercise regimens as early in the development of the disease as possible. Over the years, of course, I have had to help many patients who came to me with arthritis that had already advanced beyond the beginning stages. In such cases, I would recommend that patients begin to follow the regimens in my plan, but I would also take whatever other measures I deemed necessary to treat the intense pain and lack of mobility from which they were suffering. Even then, however, I would take the most conservative steps first before moving on to more advanced stages of care. I would begin by prescribing the least dangerous oral medications, and if those didn't help, I would carefully prescribe other medications that had a higher degree of risk associated with them. I would often combine oral medications with some form of medical care that involved external physical manipulation, such as massage therapy, osteopathy, chiropractic, physical therapy, or aquatherapy.

Only if none of those courses of treatment brought the patient significant relief would I recommend various kinds of injections, minimally invasive procedures, and finally invasive surgery. So let's take a look at the full range of medical options available to treat arthritis, beginning with over-the-counter medications, the kind you can find in any drugstore.

## ORAL MEDICATIONS: ACETAMINOPHEN

If you are still experiencing pain and discomfort after following the Arthritis Rx Plan of Stage One Care, you may want to introduce some form of oral medication into your regimen, beginning with readily available drugs that do not require a doctor's prescription. Acetaminophen (Tylenol) is a good, safe first choice for those with moderate arthritis. An analgesic (pain reliever) that was approved by the FDA over fifty years ago, acetaminophen relieves pain by elevating the pain threshold, requiring a greater amount of pain to develop before we feel it. Adults can take up to 1 gram (1,000 mg) three times a day. I caution patients to stay within this limit because excessive amounts of Tylenol can cause liver problems. Tylenol should be taken with water a half hour before or two hours after meals. To minimize stomach upset, some people like to drink milk rather than water with Tylenol. The drug takes effect in about a half hour; pain relief lasts about three to four hours.

Tylenol also comes in a time-released form that contains 650 mg of acetaminophen, so only two tablets should be taken every eight hours. Individuals must be careful to avoid taking other cold or flu remedies at the same time. Some of these preparations contain acetaminophen too, which can quickly exceed the recommended dosage. Like all drugs, Tylenol has some disadvantages. Some people report side effects such as gastrointestinal distress, fatigue, and lightheadedness. Acetaminophen, the active ingredient in Tylenol, is also available in a number of generic brands that are equally effective and generally cost less than the brand-name drug. Just be sure that the label lists acetaminophen as the primary ingredient.


## NSAIDS

Nonsteroidal anti-inflammatory drugs (NSAIDs) include the traditional medications that have been used for decades to treat arthritis, and the newer generation known as COX-2 inhibitors. I often suggest to my patients who have not responded to acetaminophen that they take ibuprofen (Motrin, Advil). Ibuprofen works by interfering with the formation of prostaglandins, substances in the body that cause inflammation and make nerves more sensitive to pain impulses. For moderate pain, arthritis patients take 200 to 400 mg of ibuprofen every four to six hours. I recommend 1,600 mg maximum a day in order to avoid kidney problems and ulcers. For best results, ibuprofen should be taken with meals. Side effects are mild in most people and include abdominal pain, indigestion, and nausea. Once again, less expensive generic brands are readily available.

There are a number of other NSAIDs that can be used as well. Each has specific advantages and disadvantages. Of these, only aspirin and Aleve are available without a prescription.

| Drug | Advantage | Disadvantage |
|------|-----------|--------------|
| Arthrotec | Most potent | High side effects; should not be taken by people with cardiac arrhythmia |
| Aspirin | High potency | High risk of ulcers |
| Lodine | Moderate potency | Moderate stomach irritation |
| Naprosyn, Aleve (naproxen) | Moderate potency | Moderate stomach irritation |
| Mobic and Relafen | Mild potency | Very mild side effects |

The prostaglandins that NSAIDs interfere with do serve a useful function by protecting the digestive tract from the deleterious effects of stomach acid. By retarding the growth of prostaglandins, NSAIDs can lead to bleeding in the stomach or the first part of the small intestines into which the stomach empties. Prolonged irritation of these areas can lead to ulcers. It is best to avoid alcohol and cigarettes when taking NSAIDs because alcohol and nicotine increase the risk of developing ulcers in these areas of the digestive system. Aspirin, which is the oldest medication for arthritis, can irritate the stomach and should not be used in high doses because of the risk of ulcers. In low doses, such as baby aspirin (81 mg) or enteric-coated doses of 325 mg, aspirin is often used as a protective measure against heart attack and stroke.

NSAIDs require careful monitoring when used by patients who take other medications, such as blood-thinning drugs, lithium, or methotrexate as part of their treatment for other conditions. Prolonged use of NSAIDs can cause kidney problems, especially in patients with diabetes. NSAIDs can also result in increased blood pressure, a risk factor for many health problems. To avoid these complications, I recommend drug holidays—no medications one day a week—during long-term use, along with blood tests to measure kidney function. Patients don't feel significantly worse as there is still plenty of medication in their system. Patients with diabetes should complete these blood tests twice a year. Patients at risk for heart disease should have an annual blood test.

However, I advise patients to avoid long-term use of NSAIDs altogether and take these drugs only in spurts during acute pain stages. My colleague Stephen A. Paget, M.D., physician in chief of the Division of Rheumatology at the Hospital for Special Surgery, also advises patients to be careful in the use of NSAIDs. He points out that there is a difference between clinically obvious and symptomatic osteoarthritis and the level of the disease that shows up on X-rays or MRIs but is "surprisingly mild." During treatment he recommends varying levels of care depending on the amount of pain, the patients' activities, and their co-morbidities (complications due to other conditions). NSAIDs are not recommended for individuals with coronary heart disease who take the anti-coagulant drug Coumadin (warfarin).

# COX-2 INHIBITORS

Because so many individuals use NSAIDs, scientists came up with a new class of drugs in the 1990s to decrease the risk of ulcers, bleeding, and perforation of the stomach or intestine. Research had shown that the NSAIDs reduce pain by inhibiting cyclooxygenase-2 (COX-2), an enzyme in the body that produces inflammation. Unfortunately, NSAIDs have a downside: They also inhibit COX-1 (the good COX), a substance that enables the stomach to protect itself against bleeding.

The new class of drugs became known as COX-2 inhibitors, because they do not inhibit COX-1, and so reduce the pain of arthritis while significantly diminishing the risk of digestive side effects including bleeding ulcers. Approved by the FDA in 1998, Celebrex was the first COX-2 inhibitor; Vioxx and Bextra soon followed. Vioxx, however, was voluntarily withdrawn from the market in 2004 after studies found that a group of individuals who had used Vioxx had a higher risk of heart attacks. Manufacturers of the other COX-2 inhibitors became concerned that their drugs might also increase this risk, and Bextra was withdrawn from the market in April 2005.

As far as COX-2 inhibitors and NSAIDs are concerned, patients must keep in mind that both can cause heart and kidney problems and must be carefully monitored when they are used. COX-2 inhibitors may increase the risk of heart attacks and strokes, as observed in several studies involving Vioxx. The manufacturers of Celebrex claim that there is no increased risk of heart attacks from their drug.

However, studies conducted by independent researchers and without the financial sponsorship of the drug companies have not been completed. Until the results of these independent analyses are available, I currently limit the use of COX-2 inhibitors to patients who have a low risk of heart disease and cannot take NSAIDs because they have ulcers. I advise against the use of COX-2 inhibitors by people with high blood pressure and those with a history of heart disease. Not only do COX-2 inhibitors increase blood pressure, but they can also increase the risk of blood clot formation, putting patients at greater risk for heart disease.

I recommend that those who take COX-2 inhibitors take a baby aspirin every day to minimize the risk of heart disease and that they take COX-2 inhibitors only in spurts. If patients must use them for six months or more, I advise them to take a drug holiday one day a week, as with NSAIDs. Individuals with diabetes should have a blood test twice a year to measure the effect of the drug on their kidneys. Other patients should have the blood test once a year. People with arthritis and rheumatoid arthritis may also use COX-2 inhibitors if everything else has failed and they still have pain. If the patient has a history of GI problems, a proton pump inhibitor drug may be needed to protect the stomach. Because of the controversy over the role of COX-2 drugs in increasing the risk of heart attack, physicians are using them less often as the initial drug to control pain. Many doctors have shifted to Mobic, Arthrotec, and Naprosyn, but we are not confident in any of these drugs anymore. As in the past, the physician and the patient in partnership have to make practical and cost-benefit decisions when a patient has persistent pain. But, clearly, COX-2 inhibitors are no longer used as they once were.

Unless we solve the problem of blood clotting and heart disease as a result of COX-2 use, the future of these drugs remains questionable. And it bears repeating that all oral medications, whether over-the-counter or prescription, carry risks with repeated use. Aspirin and ibuprofen have been shown to accelerate the breakdown of cartilage in joints if taken over a long period of time. Although this breakdown of joint cartilage is well documented, few patients are ever informed of it. This is another reason to take NSAIDs in short spurts, to avoid these kinds of complications on top of risks to the kidneys and heart.


## DOXYCYCLINE


Doxycycline is an antibiotic medicine belonging to the class called tetracyclines, and is used to treat bacterial infections such as conjunctivitis and typhus. But data in a 2005 study in *Arthritis & Rheumatism* show that doxycycline is effective in treating osteoarthritis with significant amounts of inflammation. I sometimes prescribe 100 mg of doxycycline daily for two to three months as a metalloproteinase inhibitor to decrease inflammation in arthritis patients with significant synovitis (inflammation of the synovial membrane of the joints). Metalloproteinases are enzymes involved in the repair of cartilage. In some instances of arthritis, however, they are overproduced, causing significant inflammation that can lead to further cartilage damage. Metalloproteinase inhibitors such as doxycycline play an important role in reducing inflammation and generating a cartilage-protective effect. We use it as an anti-inflammatory and not as an antibiotic in this case. Exposure to sun should be limited when on doxycycline, and it has the potential side effect of nausea.

## INTEGRATIVE CARE

One of the most important trends in arthritis treatment is the recognition that patients function at their best if they learn how to manage the stress of living with a chronic disease. To achieve this goal, an increasing number of patients work with a team of professionals from many disciplines. Besides general practice and specialist physicians who regularly treat arthritis, teams may include physical therapists, osteopaths, massage therapists, chiropractors, and acupuncturists. Whereas M.D.s and physical therapists are said to practice conventional medicine, other caregivers provide treatments that ease pain and improve quality of life but are still considered outside the realm of conventional medicine.

The area of treatment that falls outside allopathic, or conventional, medicine has been called by various names over the years. These treatment modalities were originally referred to as alternative medicine or alternative treatments. But "alternative" was felt to be somewhat pejorative, and so the term "complementary medicine" was adopted. I prefer to call these healing modalities "integrative medicine," because that term emphasizes the fact that we are using these other therapies together with conventional medical therapies, with no prejudice toward one or the other, to achieve an even better clinical effect. Just because you are undergoing massage therapy for your hip does not mean that you cannot also take anti-inflammatories, do physical therapy, follow the Arthritis Rx Exercises, or receive hylan injections. Integrative therapies are meant to stand alone or enhance effects of conventional therapies. Let's take a look at some of the most popular and most widely accepted therapeutic modalities.

## PHYSICAL THERAPY

Because physical therapists receive rigorous training in conventional medicine and have extensive knowledge of the musculoskeletal system, physicians for patients with early as well as advanced arthritis often prescribe physical therapy. By using a device called a goniometer, physical therapists evaluate the range of motion of joints, a key factor in coming up with a treatment plan. They use a variety of tests to determine muscle imbalances, flexibility, and other factors that enable the team to tailor a program to the patient's specific needs. The physical therapy program may include exercises to preserve the use of joints, maintain strength in the surrounding muscles, and help the patient continue to take part in the activities of daily living. Physical therapists use a variety of modalities: heat and cold, aquatherapy, and recreational activities, which have been described in earlier chapters.

Physical therapists use several devices to help arthritis patients cope with pain. For example, diathermy (electromagnetic waves of different frequencies) is used to deliver heat deep into the tissues. Patients with chronic pain may receive transcutaneous electrical nerve stimulation (TENS). The TENS device, which consists of a battery pack and electrodes, produces a pleasant tingling sensation and has been remarkably successful in relieving a wide range of pain and discomfort.

Physical therapists can also suggest assistive devices to make it easier for individuals with arthritis to perform household chores and activities at work. Long-handled grippers, for example, are designed to grasp and retrieve out-of-reach objects. Physical therapists can also teach patients how to use proper body mechanics to get in and out of cars, chairs, and bathtubs, or how to lift objects to minimize stress on joints. Physical therapy can take place at a hospital, a physical therapy office, or a patient's home. A physical therapist who has completed the orthopedic specialty and has a certificate or a doctorate in physical therapy and specializes in treating arthritis is a good choice.

## OSTEOPATHY

In addition to physical therapists, many individuals are using the services of other professionals, such as osteopaths, who provide body-based procedures. Osteopaths believe that the body has self-healing mechanisms and that one way to release them is by therapeutic manipulation of the bones, joints, and soft tissues. Therapeutic manipulation of the body has ancient roots: Hippocrates used it in the fifth century B.C., but it was not until the birth of osteopathy in the 1890s that formalized programs were developed. Today, osteopathic medical schools provide rigorous education in the basic sciences as well as all aspects of human health, similar to allopathic medical schools. Osteopaths learn to use their hands to identify the areas where the patient is experiencing pain. Then they apply one or more of thirty different manual techniques to restore the disordered body framework to optimal mechanical and structural ease. The goal is to enhance overall bodily movement and the function of the nervous and circulatory systems, and to improve nutrition and drainage to tissues by way of assisting the body's healing processes.

Osteopathic techniques fall into three general categories. Osteopaths have developed many soft tissue techniques to affect the mechanical and neural dysfunctions of the body's muscular and connective tissues. They use manipulative techniques to improve mobility of the joints and neural distortion and to restore normal fluid dynamics. Finally, specific joint techniques include subtle methods to repair joint dysfunction and restore mobility and function to a particular region of the body. Many of the techniques are named after their founders, such as Greenman muscle-energy and Jones counterstrain. Other common techniques include myofascial release, and cranial-sacral therapy (formally known as osteopathy in the cranial field). I have seen great benefits to my patients with spine and hip arthritis from talented osteopathic physicians and colleagues, such as Dr. Brian Waldron and Dr. David Gentile, both of New York. Osteopaths generally have the initials D.O., for Doctor of Osteopathy, after their name.

## CHIROPRACTIC

Chiropractors give special attention to the physiological and biochemical aspects of the body, "including structural, spinal, musculoskeletal, neurological, vascular, nutritional, emotional, and environmental relationships," according to the American Chiropractic Association. The practices and procedures that chiropractors employ include the adjustment and manipulation of the joints and adjacent tissues, particularly the spinal column. Chiropractic is a drug-free, non-surgical science, so chiropractors don't prescribe pharmaceuticals or invasive surgery.

The roots of chiropractic care can be traced back to China and Greece in the fifth and fourth centuries B.C. Hippocrates (*ca* 460 to *ca* 377 B.C.) published texts describing the importance of chiropractic care, writing, "Get knowledge of the spine, for this is the requisite for many diseases." In this country, the practice of spinal manipulation began to gain acceptance during the late nineteenth century, and the profession was officially founded in 1895 by Daniel David Palmer in Davenport, Iowa.

Chiropractors now provide most of the manipulative therapy in the U.S. Although there have been numerous trials of manipulative therapy for back pain patients, there have been few studies of its effectiveness in treating arthritis. However, I have seen my patients with lower-back arthritis benefit greatly from gentle chiropractic manipulations with excellent practitioners such as Dr. Carol Goldstein, based in Manhattan. Accredited chiropractors have the initials D.C., for Doctor of Chiropractic, after their name. I caution patients with neck arthritis to avoid aggressive manipulations, because they may be at risk for stroke or spinal cord injuries.

## MASSAGE THERAPY

As I discussed earlier, medical massage is an important component of many patients' treatment plans. During a massage, a therapist manipulates the body's soft
tissues—the muscles, skin, and tendons—using fingertips, hands, and fists. Massage
therapists as well as physical therapists can perform massages, of which there are
several types. Swedish is the most common form, consisting of long smooth strokes
and kneading movements along the skin. All parts of the body can be worked during
this type of massage.

"Unlike Swedish massage, which concentrates on the soft tissues near the surface of the skin," says Rick Sharpell, a talented massage therapist in New York City,
"deep massage uses slow, heavy strokes to create direct pressure and friction on the
muscles. The target of this massage is the deep muscle tissue. Some massage therapists combine these techniques to help patients [achieve relief] with specific muscle
groups."

Although many patients report positive results from massage, there have been
no definitive studies of their impact on the pain of arthritis patients.


## ACUPUNCTURE

Acupuncture has become one of the most popular therapies in the U.S. The National Institutes of Health estimate that more than 15 million individuals in this
country have tried the needle therapy for conditions ranging from arthritis and
asthma to nausea and chronic pain. The practice of inserting thin needles into specific body points to improve health and well-being originated in China more than
two thousand years ago.

The Chinese believe that an essential life energy called *chi* flows through the
body along invisible channels, or meridians. When the flow of chi is blocked or out

of balance, illness or pain results. Stimulation of specific points along the meridians can correct the flow of chi and block pain or restore health.

Western scientists don't know exactly how acupuncture works. They suspect, however, that the meridians correspond to areas called trigger points that are rich in nerve endings. They believe that stimulating these pressure points with needles produces a cascade of chemicals in the muscles, spinal cord, and brain that releases endorphins, the body's natural pain-killing substances.

A 2004 scientific study published in *Annals of Internal Medicine* found that acupuncture relieves knee arthritis symptoms. Relief is often temporary and treatments must be repeated. For best results, choose a therapist who is licensed and/or a graduate of a respected school of acupuncture, and someone who is willing to work with your physician. About ten thousand acupuncturists currently practice in the U.S.; most are regulated by the state in which they reside. About four thousand physicians have completed a recognized acupuncture training program.

Although experts agree that acupuncture, massage therapy, and other treatment programs won't cure arthritis, these treatments add another dimension to the management of pain.

Of the common alternatives to conventional medical care for arthritis, only massage therapy and acupuncture have so far been proven effective in clinical trials. There is other, if less rigorous, medical evidence for the value of osteopathic and chiropractic care, however, and I have seen many patients helped by both of them. Based on my experience in working with patients, I have determined that acupuncture works well for knee, wrist-hand, and foot-ankle arthritis. Although a recent study has shown that acupuncture is effective in treating knee arthritis, clinical studies have proven that it does not work for lower-back arthritis. For in-depth information on lower-back arthritis, I advise you to refer to my first book, *Back Rx*. For hip and lower-back arthritis, I have seen better results with osteopathy. Chiropractic treatments also work well for lower-back arthritis, and therapeutic massage works for arthritis of the neck, lower back, and hip.

And I have anecdotal evidence that aquatherapy works well for knee arthritis. One of my relatives, who is sixty-four, is an electrical engineer and has suffered for years from knee arthritis that was caused by a cricket injury he sustained in his twenties. About seven years ago, I convinced him to start aquatherapy, and he now does it five days a week. He does not follow any of the other aspects of my Arthritis Rx Plan besides aquatherapy, and yet he claims that this one simple activity has kept up his mobility and minimized his pain despite a significantly arthritic knee.

---

## WEB SITES FOR SOME LEADING ORGANIZATIONS OF INTEGRATIVE MEDICINE

| | |
|---|---|
| American Osteopathic Association | osteopathic.org |
| American Massage Therapy Association | amta.org |
| American Association of Oriental Medicine (acupuncture) | aaom.org |
| American Chiropractic Association | amerchiro.org |
| American College of Rheumatology | rheumatology.org |
| American Academy of Physical Medicine and Rehabilitation | aapmr.org |
| American Association of Orthopaedic Surgeons | aaos.org |

# CHAPTER THIRTEEN

# STAGE THREE CARE:
# MINIMALLY INVASIVE,
# NON-SURGICAL PROCEDURES

For arthritic pain that does not respond to Stage Two care, patients may bene-fit from a variety of procedures that can be performed in the doctor's office. They involve various kinds of injections, but the patient can return home the same day and no anesthesia is involved.

## HYLAN (HYALURONIC ACID)

In Chapter One, I mentioned that the joints have an ally in their battle to reduce de-structive friction, a liquid called synovial fluid that lubricates the joint like motor oil and allows great freedom of movement. Synovial fluid is found in the bursa, a small, sac-shaped membrane in the knee and many other joints. One of the principal en-zymes that make up synovial fluid is hyaluronic acid (HA). During advanced arthri-tis, the synovial fluid of the affected joints loses as much as one-third to two-thirds of its HA. A synthetic form of HA called hylan, made from rooster combs or bacterial cultures, can be injected into the joints to revitalize the synovial fluid and recapture smooth, pain-free movement. (Those who are allergic to eggs or poultry must use the bacterial form.) This therapy has been used in Europe and Asia for many years. In 1997 the FDA approved hylan as a treatment for arthritis of the knee, but now it is being extensively used "off label" (applications not originally specified by the FDA) by physicians in the U.S. to treat arthritis of the hip, shoulder, ankle, and hand.

I have studied the use of hylan extensively in clinical trials involving over 2,000 knees, 1,800 hips, 80 shoulders, 50 ankles, 25 toes, and 20 hands. The early results have been quite promising. Our research shows that 50 percent of the patients with knee arthritis reported significant pain relief one year after injections. Injections of hylan are most effective when preceded by joint lavage. In this procedure, a physician repeatedly injects saline solution into the joint space to flush out the debris and then withdraws it before administering the hyaluronic acid. Our research indicates that combining these techniques decreased pain more and lasted longer than either treatment alone—the success rate increased to 80 percent. Results improve further if the lavage and injections are combined with proper exercise programs such as Arthritis Rx and modalities such as icing.

Similar promising results occurred in the off-label use of hylan for the treatment of hip arthritis. Both studies were published in peer-reviewed journals in 2003. Results for shoulder and ankle arthritis have also been promising. Four hylan formulations, called viscosupplements, are commercially available. One is crosslinked (Synvisc), whereas the other three are not (Supartz, Orthovisc, and Hyalgan), but there is no evidence that any one brand is better than the others. Those with severe arthritis and obesity don't do as well with hylan treatments.

There is early evidence that hylan may slow the progression of arthritis and protect cartilage. However, hylan combined with joint lavage and the Arthritis Rx Plan exhibit tremendous synergy, and the success rate goes up exponentially. Arthritis exercises and an anti-inflammatory diet also slow the progression. The vast majority of patients with mild to moderate arthritis who combine these regimens and treatments will remain mobile and pain-free and avoid the need for surgical intervention.

## CORTISONE INJECTIONS

Corticosteroids are a family of drugs that include cortisol (hydrocortisone, or just cortisone)—an adrenal hormone found naturally in the body—as well as synthetic drugs. Natural cortisone is produced by the body's adrenal glands, and is normally released into the bloodstream when your body is under stress. It is relatively short acting. Injectible cortisone is synthetically produced and has many different trade names, but is closely related to the body's own product. Although natural and synthetic corticosteroids are both potent anti-inflammatory compounds, the synthetics exert a stronger effect. Some oral forms of corticosteroids are used to treat autoimmune and inflammatory conditions, including asthma, bursitis, and Crohn's disease, as well as severe allergic reactions.

The most significant difference between natural and synthetic cortisone is that the synthetic form is not injected into the bloodstream but into a particular area of inflammation, such as the knee or hip joint. Synthetic cortisone is also designed to act more potently and for a longer period of time—days instead of minutes.

An injection of a cortisone is sometimes indicated if the arthritis patient has acute pain in a swollen joint. A possible side effect is temporary swelling at the injection site, a "cortisone flare," whereby the injected cortisone crystallizes and can cause a brief period of pain. This lasts a day or two at most and can be treated by icing the injected area. The efficacy of cortisone injections for chronic arthritis pain is limited, so I limit these injections to a maximum of three a year for patients who have an acute arthritis flare-up that causes a swollen joint. The use of cortisone should also be limited because excessive use can lead to cartilage damage. Some patients with diabetes may have a transient increase in their blood-sugar levels, which they should monitor closely. On the whole, I have seen great benefits from cortisone for treating flare-ups but very limited short-term benefits for chronic arthritis patients who don't present with acute flare-ups. Cortisone injections must be performed by a physician, but they represent a minimal risk and a conservative approach to managing pain and regaining full range of motion in patients with occasional acute flare-ups.

Injections of hylan must also be performed by a physician, with only a minor risk of side effects, such as slight swelling or bruising. When combined with the proper exercise regimen, injections represent attractive options for patients with moderate arthritis who are not obese. Therapies such as hylan will continue to improve and to be used in a wider number of joints as time goes by.

# CHAPTER FOURTEEN

# STAGE FOUR CARE: SURGICAL INTERVENTION

There are instances when knee and hip pain caused by arthritis don't respond to weight loss, physical therapy, and other conservative measures. Over time, pain medications may prove ineffective. At that juncture, many patients consider surgical interventions. My colleague, Thomas P. Sculco, M.D., surgeon in chief at the Hospital for Special Surgery in New York and a pioneering orthopedic surgeon, explained: "Surgical interventions have come a long way in the past twenty-five years. Advances in techniques, technology, infection control, and anesthesia have made a significant difference in joint replacement surgery. We can do more today to help people with arthritis live fuller, more active lives."

The most common reason for having a hip or knee replaced is pain.

"Pain is relative," says Dr. Sculco. "A thirty-five-year-old male may consider surgery when the pain begins to interfere with his ability to engage in recreational sports. On the other hand, a seventy-year-old woman may not consider surgery even though her pain is so intense that she cannot walk across a room." To help patients reach a decision, Dr. Sculco suggests that patients consider the impact of arthritis on their lives. Does the pain of arthritis prevent them from sleeping? Have they stopped taking walks, visiting friends, and doing other activities? Do they have difficulty getting out of a chair or climbing stairs? An increasing number of people are opting for joint replacement. About 326,000 knees and 168,000 hip joints were replaced in 2001, according to the National Center for Health Statistics.

## TOTAL KNEE REPLACEMENT

The largest joint in the body, the knee is formed where the lower part of the thighbone (femur) joins the upper part of the shinbone (tibia) and the kneecap (patella). The knee has three compartments: the medial (inside), the lateral (outside), and the kneecap. In addition, the knee has two special cartilages called the lateral meniscus and the medial meniscus, which act as shock absorbers. Two ligaments—the anterior cruciate and the posterior cruciate—contribute to knee stability. Arthritis robs the knee of its ability to glide, causing stiffness, limiting mobility, and making some knees lock or click. Pain usually develops in the inside part of the knee, but may be felt in the front or back of the knee as well. As cartilage is worn away, some people become more knock-kneed or bowlegged.

When only some of the joint is damaged, an orthopedic surgeon may be able to repair or replace just the damaged parts. When the entire joint is affected, a total joint replacement is done. In a standard total knee replacement, the damaged areas of the thighbone, shinbone, and kneecap are removed and replaced with a prosthesis (artificial joint). The ends of the remaining bones are smoothed and reshaped to accommodate the prosthesis. The orthopedic surgeon either uses bone cement— similar to what a dentist uses for artificial teeth—to secure the prosthesis in place or implants with uneven, rough ends that allow new bone to grow into the implant.

Total knee replacement is recommended for a wide variety of patients because it can dramatically improve the quality of life for a person with debilitating pain. In the past, the procedure was typically performed on older adults, but now it is considered for adults of all ages. Young, physically active patients are candidates, thanks to better implants. Patients in their forties and fifties were reluctant to undergo knee replacement surgery because they feared that their artificial joints would wear out, making another knee replacement necessary. The initial knee prostheses were made of metal and plastic. Although the metal was highly polished and the polyethylene was intended to be wear-resistant, the daily rubbing of these surfaces against each other during normal movements created tiny particles of debris. After many years, these particles sometimes damaged the surrounding bone and loosened the prosthesis.

"Today improved materials, designs, and manufacturing methods have helped overcome the wear and tear problem," says Dr. Sculco. "Studies show that a knee replacement now lasts at least twenty years in about 90 percent of those who get them." In addition to prostheses made of metal and plastic, there are now three other types of surfaces: metal-on-metal, ceramic-on-polyethylene, and ceramic-on-ceramic. Unlike the clay ceramic used in pottery, the ceramic used in knee replacement is highly durable because it is made from aluminum or zirconium chemically combined with oxygen.

The prostheses come in a variety of designs that take into account the patient's age, weight, activity level, and overall health. As a result, these artificial joints help replicate the knee's natural ability to produce smooth movements. The artificial knees are held in place by either bone cement or an uncemented implant. In most cases, uncemented implants are used because they are less likely to loosen over time and impair the stability of the joint. Patients who have poor-quality bone, such as older women, usually receive cemented joints.

Like any surgery, total knee-joint replacement involves certain risks including infection and complications from anesthesia. In the rare case that an infection spreads to the new joint and does not clear up with antibiotic treatment, the joint must be replaced. This usually involves two surgeries—one to remove the infected joint and another to insert the new joint.

To reduce the risk of infection, orthopedic surgeons like Dr. Sculco operate in "space suits." The operating rooms at the Hospital for Special Surgery are also equipped with a special laminar airflow system to remove bacteria. Anesthesia has improved to the point where an epidural catheter—a small tube inserted into the patient's back—is used during surgery and is kept in place for one to two days to help with pain control during recovery.

Total joint replacement surgery takes one-and-a-half to two hours. Patients go home after two to three days, and in three to six weeks they are generally back to their daily activities. They complete physical therapy in the hospital or office and at home.

Whenever possible, of course, we recommend a minimally invasive form of knee surgery. Instead of the traditional six- to twelve-inch-long incision used in standard total knee replacement, some surgeons now perform the surgery through a four- to five-inch incision. The advantage of a minimally invasive technique is that it decreases trauma to muscles, tissues, and tendons. Patients have less pain after surgery and go home more quickly.

## TOTAL HIP REPLACEMENT

The largest ball-and-socket joint, the hip, bears the body's full weight. The ball of the joint, the top of the thighbone (femoral head) moves within the hollow socket (acetabulum) of the pelvis. The thighbone and the pelvic bone are separated by cartilage. When the cartilage is damaged by arthritis, the hip becomes stiff and movement is painful. The same criteria for knee replacement generally apply to hip replacement—pain and loss of function. Good candidates for total hip replacement are patients who have not received relief from more conservative therapies. The good news is that hips damaged by arthritis are also benefiting from advances in surgery. Minimal incision—three to five inches—rather than the ten- to twelve-inch incisions in standard hip replacement have decreased soreness, according to Dr. Sculco, and patients are able to get up and move around sooner.

Hip replacement surgery is now one of the most common joint replacement surgeries. The procedure used to be reserved for people older than sixty who were less active and therefore less likely to wear out their artificial joints. But improved technology has made stronger and longer-lasting artificial joints that are more feasible for a younger, more active person. Younger people still face the possibility of repeated surgery after twenty years as wear breaks down the artificial hip joint, but revision surgery—although more technically difficult—has improved. (There continue to be exciting advances in the quality and durability of hip replacement materials, and I'll have more to say on this at the end of the book.)

Total hip replacement surgery usually takes two to three hours, and patients are encouraged to sit up later that day. They go home after three or four days and continue their exercises. During the procedure, the orthopedic surgeon cuts away the ball part of the joint, replacing it with a ball attached to a stem that is wedged into a hollowed-out space in the thighbone. Damaged cartilage and bone are removed from the socket and the ball-like component is inserted into the socket. Hip replacements may be cemented or uncemented. Patients complete strengthening and mobility exercises in the hospital and use a cane at first.

Blood clots are a risk in any joint surgery because of decreased movement of the leg. Blood-thinning medications and improved surgical techniques have decreased this risk. As a result, the odds of a successful hip replacement surgery are in your favor. Studies show that the chance of your hip replacement lasting twenty years, when done by experienced hip replacement surgeons, is 90 percent.


## ARTHROSCOPY


A minimally invasive surgical technique, arthroscopy, is now used to treat a range of conditions affecting joints, including arthritis. My colleague Struan H. Coleman, M.D., Ph.D., who specializes in sports medicine at the Hospital for Special Surgery, explains that in using the arthroscopic technique, the orthopedic surgeon can smooth defects or remove small pieces of loose tissue that may contribute to arthritis of the knee and lead to symptoms such as clicking or locking. During the procedure, the surgeon makes tiny incisions in the affected joint and then inserts a tiny camera and fiber optics to light the interior space. Pictures obtained with the camera are then projected onto the screen in the operating room, enabling the surgeon to get multiple views inside the joint.

After inserting the instruments through the tiny skin incisions, the surgeon removes cartilage fragments and flushes the joint with saline. The incisions may be closed with stitches if necessary. The entire procedure takes about an hour and the patient goes home the same day. Physical therapy helps the patient recover and regain range of motion within a few weeks.

Hip arthroscopy has been slower to evolve than arthroscopy of the knee and shoulder because the hip joint is located much deeper in the body and is harder to access. Currently, the role of arthroscopic surgery in arthritis is quite limited. It is used for small cartilage lesions with techniques available for microfractures. The number of patients who qualify for these procedures is fewer than 1 percent of the arthritic population. I caution my patients to keep in mind that degenerative meniscus tears of the knee and degenerative labral tears of the hip rarely cause pain and should be left alone.


## RESURFACING


One alternative to total hip replacement is a procedure called hip resurfacing, which is currently undergoing clinical trials and should soon be approved by the FDA. Unlike the prosthesis used in total hip replacement, which is made to replace the femoral head, resurfacing allows the head to be preserved and reshaped. The resurfaced bone is then capped with a metal prosthesis. Like total hip replacement, the socket is fitted with a prosthesis. Not everyone is a candidate for resurfacing, according to Dr. Edwin Su at the Hospital for Special Surgery, who has significant experience with this new technology. The femoral head may be too damaged to hold the resurfacing component, and good bone stock is also required, Dr. Su advises.

## OSTEOTOMY

Patients who have moderate arthritis that is confined to one part of the knee make good candidates for a procedure called osteotomy. Good candidates are those who have limited damage to the joint. During osteotomy, the orthopedic surgeon removes some of the diseased bone and tissue and realigns the knee. This takes the pressure off the arthritic area and places weight bearing on relatively uninvolved portions of the knee joint. The advantage of this type of surgery is that the patient's own knee joint is retained and could potentially provide many years of pain-free activity. The disadvantage is a longer rehabilitation course—six to twelve months in some cases—and the possibility that arthritis could develop in the newly aligned knee.

Today a hip or knee replacement is likely to last twenty years, but in the future, replacements may last even longer as researchers and orthopedic surgeons continue to offer more options in prostheses and surgical techniques.

# EPILOGUE:

# THE FUTURE OF ARTHRITIS CARE

So much of what I have offered in this book consists of prescriptions for basic healthful living that even if you were magically healed of arthritis tomorrow, you would do well to follow it anyway. And although I said earlier that there is currently no cure for arthritis, we are coming closer to a time when it may be possible to halt the progression of the disease. Before I leave you, let me discuss for a moment the future of arthritis care both from my own perspective and from the viewpoints of some of the leading researchers in the field.

According to Dr. Clifford Colwell, Jr., who heads the orthopedic research effort at the Scripps Clinic in San Diego, the first thing we need is much more research to learn exactly what happens on the cellular level at the onset of arthritis. "Treatment will ultimately depend on discovering the etiology [cause or origin of the disease]. If it turns out that arthritis is based on genetics, then it will respond to a genetic approach." Determining the precise cause will lead to the development of targeted technologies for treating arthritis. In March 2005, together with my wife, my parents, and other family members, I founded the Vad Foundation with the mission of educating disadvantaged children and funding basic science studies evaluating what causes arthritis. Once we discover that, our ability to treat the disease will improve exponentially. (To date the foundation has funded two scholarships for inner-city youths and one basic research study on arthritis.)

In the near term, arthritis care will be focusing on newer composite materials that can allow artificial hip or knee replacements to last forty to fifty years. "The best approach is a combination of improved mechanical design and new materials," says Prof. Subhash Risbud, Professor of Materials Science at the University of California at Davis and a Visiting Professor of Chemical Engineering at Stanford University in the Center on Polymer Interfaces and Macromolecular Assemblies. Hip replacements essentially consist of a stem and a ball-and-socket assembly attached to the bones in the hip. In the past these parts have been made of metal, polyethylene, ceramic, or some combination of these. The problem with metal-on-metal replacements is that the metal parts wear down by scraping against each other and throwing off tiny fragments—"often in the form of nanoscale particles or debris," as Prof. Risbud calls them. Sometimes these nanoparticles find their way into the bloodstream, and if the metal involved is cobalt or titanium, for instance, that can be toxic for the patient. Polyethylene also wears down because it's too soft. Alumina- and zirconia-based ceramic implants are safer, but ceramics tend to be more brittle than metals and break when too much stress is placed on them. For several years now, ceramics researchers have developed a way of toughening the ceramic. Zirconia-toughened alumina (ZTA) is considerably higher in strength and toughness than standard alumina (aluminum oxide) as a result of the precipitation-induced toughening achieved by microstructures of fine zirconia particles dispersed uniformly throughout the alumina. This creates a ceramic similar to that used in mechanically demanding applications both at conventional and high temperatures. Further, the improved wear and tribological properties of these deliberately engineered ceramics—their ability to withstand friction—can be expected to add many years of use to hip replacement joints.

"Whereas metal components wear down at the rate of roughly 0.1 to 0.4 mm per year," Prof. Risbud says, "toughened ceramics wear at rates as low as 0.002 mm per year. And as the risk of brittle failure keeps getting lower with better ceramic structures and improved design, the confidence in hip replacement components will keep increasing." Further, he has every reason to believe that with the advent of newer ceramic processing technologies, implant production will become cheaper and quicker over the next few years.

As astonishing as that progress seems, it's barely the tip of the iceberg, according to Joseph Buckwalter, M.D., the head of the Department of Orthopaedic Surgery at the University of Iowa Hospitals and Clinics, and one of the two or three leading authorities on arthritis in the world. In his opinion, the most promising emerging treatments for arthritis are "local therapies." What that deceptively simple phrase means is that instead of continuing to use systemic therapies—endlessly prescribing pills for arthritis that have unintended consequences for the entire body, including kidney problems, heart disease, and ulcers—we can treat the disease locally with little or no impact outside the treatment area. Dr. Buckwalter favors "intra-articular treatments"—the use of hylan, collagens, antioxidants, growth factors, and other local therapies that can be applied in a closely controlled manner. He believes that correcting mechanical abnormalities may also be of benefit to slow or reverse the process of joint degeneration.

The logical extension of Dr. Buckwalter's thinking is the increased use of targeted biologic therapies. These will include using stem cells taken from your own body and cultured in gels that will last longer than hylan, then injected back into the arthritic joint. Dr. John Brekke of Tissue Engineering Consultants of Duluth, Minnesota, has pioneered development of these slow-release gels utilizing hylan. These gels can also be combined with growth factors, synthetic materials that will not only grow cartilage but even stimulate the production of proper joint fluid. (Because the stem cells are taken from your body and not embryos, you can utilize them without government interference.) The biotech company I started in 2001, called Mobitech, is running trials of new gels combined with stem cells for reducing pain and markedly slowing down the progression of arthritis. And I am not alone; perhaps a dozen other biotech companies from around the country and the world are now competing to develop these new technologies.

We will soon be able to apply these technological developments not only in arthritic joints but in the vertebrae as well. There are already data to show that stem cells injected into the spinal disks will keep them from dehydrating and degenerating further. Tissue engineers, who work with different types of cells to grow new cartilage and other essential elements of the joints, such as synovial fluid or the shock-absorbing gels of spinal disks, are pioneering natural biologic treatments to replace the artificial technologies of metal and ceramics. My colleague Dr. Tae Ho Kim, a plastic surgeon and a talented tissue engineer in the area of arthritis research at the University of Southern California, predicts that within a decade or two, biologic intervention therapies will become the gold standard for treating arthritis.

The ultimate goal is early diagnosis and early intervention. If we can take charge of the disease early enough, before the disk or the cartilage wears out, we will go a long way to stopping arthritis in its tracks. If we were to consider the state-of-the-art treatments that exist today as the first generation of arthritis medicine, then the next generation of care would include some of the new technologies I have just outlined and more. It is feasible that within the next few years we will have a true COX-2 inhibitor that will relieve pain efficiently without problems of increased blood clotting and the risk of heart disease. We could also see another kind of oral medication that would limit cartilage breakdown. A number of companies are currently working to develop these kinds of disease-modifying arthritis drugs.

The third generation of arthritis treatments would combine synthetic gels with stem cells and growth factors not just to protect the cartilage but also to generate new cartilage and joint fluid. Researchers are also working on a time-released injectible gel that will actually grow bone inside the socket. We will increasingly see hybrids of artificial materials and biologic substances that will grow organic material over and around the artificial replacements to better bond them to the body.

And the fourth generation of developments would consist of gene therapy that will allow us to turn on cells to generate their own cartilage, synovial fluid, and even the gel of spinal disks. We will not just stop the loss of bone and cartilage in arthritis but completely reverse it.

Although we will see large numbers of people in our population learning to manage arthritis over the next three decades, as society ages and life spans grow longer, we will also see the emergence of promising new arthritis therapies that will eliminate pain, restore mobility, slow down or stop the progression of arthritis, and even potentially reverse the disease. The future of arthritis therapies is bright. Ultimately it is the people who will benefit with a vastly improved quality of life well into their golden years.

# APPENDIX:

# WEB RESOURCES

## ESSENTIAL INFORMATION

Arthritis Foundation: **arthritis.org**

Our book Web site and information on Arthritis Rx supplements: **zingerflex.com**

## PHYSICIAN INFORMATION

American Academy of Orthopaedic Surgeons: **aaos.org**

American Academy of Physical Medicine and Rehabilitation: **aapmr.org**

American College of Rheumatology: **rheumatology.org**

Gosden Robinson Early Arthritis Center (E.A.C.) at the Hospital for Special Surgery: **hss.edu**

## INTEGRATIVE CARE

American Association of Oriental Medicine (acupuncture): **aaom.org**

American Chiropractic Association: **amerchiro.org**

American Massage Therapy Association: **amta.org**

American Osteopathic Association: **osteopathic.org**

American Physical Therapy Association: **apta.org**

National Center for Complementary and Alternative Medicine Clearinghouse:
**nccam.nih.gov**

National Institute of Arthritis and Muscular Skeletal and Skin Diseases:
**niams.nih.gov**


## SPECIALIZED SITES FOR ARTHRITIS
## OF THE OTHER JOINTS

*Wrist and hand*

American Society for Surgery of the Hand: **assh.org**


*Foot and ankle*

American Podiatric Medical Association: **apma.org**

American Orthopaedic Foot & Ankle Society: **aofas.org**


*Shoulder*

American Shoulder and Elbow Surgeons: **ases-assn.org**


*Neck*

American Academy of Physical Medicine and Rehabilitation: **aapmr.org**

Physiatric Association of Spine, Sports and Occupational Rehabilitation
**aapmr.org/passor.htm**

North American Spine Society: **spine.org**

# INDEX

eating on the go, 107–8
eating out, 92–93
EFAs (essential fatty acids), 62
EGCG (epigallocatechin gallate), 87
eggs, 80–81, 104–5
Ehlers-Danlos Syndrome, 31
eicosanoids, 63
eicosapentaenoic acid (EPA), 77, 78, 86
elimination diets, 77, 82
Enbrel, 60
endurance, slowing arthritis, 38
energy bars, 62, 68, 70–71
environmental factors impact, 61
EPA (eicosapentaenoic acid), 77, 78, 86
epigallocatechin gallate (EGCG), 87
essential fatty acids (EFAs), 62
estrogen factor, 29
etiology, 217
exercises (Arthritis Rx)
    activities for, 44, 54, 104
    importance of, 6, 7–8, 20, 54–55
    joints (non-weight bearing) exercises, 179–88, 224
    Series A exercises (return to movement), 8, 40, 43, 125–44
    Series B exercises (resuming full activity), 8, 40, 43, 145–62
    Series C exercises (into the fast lane), 8, 43, 163–78
    slowing arthritis development, 38–44
    See also Arthritis Rx Plan; diet; weekly sampler

FABERE (Flexion, Abduction, External Rotation, and Extension), 131–32, 135
fat, 59, 66
fiber, 72, 73–74, 83, 84, 85, 89, 91
Fierce (Uneven) Posture, 177
"fight or flight" response, 41

Fingers to Toes Stretch, 136, 155
fish oil supplements, 78, 80
flavonoids, 64, 86, 89
flaxseed, 62, 63, 65, 86
Flaxseed Toast, 117–18
Flexibility Prayer, 141
flexibility, slowing arthritis, 38, 40
Flexion, Abduction, External Rotation, and Extension (FABERE), 131–32, 135
food allergies, 82
Food and Drug Administration (FDA), 69, 75, 79, 83, 101, 102, 206
foods, recommended, 63, 65, 67–72, 82–92
Foot and Ankle Exercise, 188
foot/ankle arthritis, 179, 181–82, 185, 224
Framingham Osteoarthritis Study, 44, 179
free radicals, 61–62, 75, 87, 88
fruits, 64, 65, 67, 68, 72, 73, 74, 75, 76, 107
future of arthritis care, 9, 217–21

GAIT (Glucosamine/ chondroitin Arthritis Intervention Trial), 11, 98–99
Garlic and Ginger Greens, 118
Garlic-Ginger Salmon Fillets, 118–19
gene therapy, 217, 220–21
Gentile, David, 200
Genzyme Corporation, 182
ginger, 3, 10–11, 53, 55, 65, 86, 98, 99–100, 104
Ginger and Garlic Greens, 118
Ginger-Garlic Salmon Fillets, 118–19
glenohumeral joint, 180, 181
glucosamine, 10, 11, 53, 55, 98–99, 100, 104
Glucosamine/chondroitin Arthritis Intervention Trial (GAIT), 11, 98–99
Glucosamine Unum in Die Efficacy (GUIDE) Trial, 11, 99

glucose, 59, 73
glutathione, 84–85
Goldstein, Carol, 200
Good Manufacturing Practice (GMP), 102, 104
gout, 4, 80, 89
granola, 71
grapes, 73, 86–87
Grape Tomatoes & Tuna, Brown Rice, 121
Greens, Ginger and Garlic, 118
Greens Sautéed in Olive Oil and Garlic, 119–20
green tea, 65, 87
GUIDE (Glucosamine Unum in Die Efficacy) Trial, 11, 99

Hamstring Stretch Lying Down, 170
Hamstring Stretch Seated, 172
Hand Exercise, 186
hand/wrist arthritis, 179–80, 185, 224
Harvard Medical School, 59, 60
Hatha yoga, 41
health-care practitioner, 45–47, 52
heart disease, 11, 58–59, 61, 67, 76, 80, 86, 88, 89, 90, 194, 195, 196
heat therapy, 15
heavy physical labor factor, 30–31
hemochromatosis, 31
Herberden's nodes, 26
heredity factor, 26
herperidin, 88
Hip Hikers, 135
Hippocrates, 57, 199, 200
Hippocratic oath, 51
hips
    arthritis in, 25, 26–27, 32
    musculoskeletal system, 21
    replacement, 212–13, 215, 218–19
"history and physical," 32–33, 34
homocysteine, 78, 89

227

Hospital for Special Surgery (HSS), 5, 24, 34, 182, 183, 194, 209, 211–12, 213, 214, 223
Hundred, The, 164
Hyalgan, 206
"hydrogenated" caution, 66, 71
hylan (hyaluronic acid) injections, 5–6, 180, 181, 182, 183, 205–7, 208
hypermobility disorders, 31

ibuprofen (Motrin, Advil), 14, 15, 193
ice therapy, 15
iliotibial band (ITB) stretches, 132–34
Indiana University, 38
inflammation and arthritis, 10
inflammation and diet, 58–65
ingredients, list of, 69–70
injuries from contact sports, 31–32
insulin, 59, 73, 88
integrative (complementary) care, 46–47, 197–205, 224
Intermediate Abdominal Crunch, 148
Intermediate Abdominal Crunch with Leg Flexed, 150
Intermediate Back Extension, 156–57
Intermediate Hip Hikes, 154–55
Intermediate Locust Posture, 156
"intra-articular treatments," 219

Jensen, Bernard, 83
John Paul II (Pope), 5
joint lavage, 5, 6
jointline tenderness, 33
joint replacements, 5, 6, 209–13, 218–19
joints, musculoskeletal system, 19–21
joints (non-weight bearing) exercises, 179–88, 224. *See also* exercises
*Journal of Neurological and Orthopedic Medical Surgery,* 77

Journal of Nutrition, 86

kale, 62, 63, 65, 74, 85–86
Kim, Tae Ho, 220
kiwi fruit, 87–88
knee-extension machine caution, 40
knees
  arthritis in, 27, 30, 31–32
  musculoskeletal system, 21
  replacement, 210–12, 215, 218
Knee to Chest, 129–30
Knee to Chest on All Fours, 176
Knee to Chest with Feet Flexed, 149

label reading importance, 68–72
*Lancet, The,* 53, 98
Legg Calve-Perthes disease, 31
ligaments and joints, 20, 21
liniments, 15–16
linoleic acid, 62, 63, 86
lipid peroxidation, 64
"local therapies," 219
Locust Posture, 136–37
Lodine, 193
Lou Gehrig's disease, 62
Lumbar Rotation Double Knee, 132–33
Lumbar Rotation Single Knee, 134
Lumbar Rotation with Leg Crossed, 152–53
lycopene, 90

macular degeneration, 67
magnetic resonance imaging (MRI), 34
management of arthritis, 3–4, 4–5, 7, 8
Mango and Strawberry Chutney, Spicy, 120–21
massage therapy, 9, 46, 181, 201, 202, 203, 224
Mediterranean Diet, 88
melons, 85
meniscus in knee, 21, 31–32, 33

mercury (methylmercury) in fish, 78–79
metabolic disorders factor, 31
methylsulfonylmethane (MSM), 101
minerals, 64
mineral water, 65, 90
minimally invasive, non-surgical procedures (Stage Three care), 45, 51, 52, 205–8
Mobic, 193, 196
mobility, pain-free, 19–20, 25–26, 51
Mobitech, 219–20
monosodium glutamate (MSG), 70, 71, 92
monounsaturated fats, 82, 83
Morning Tea, 120
MRI (magnetic resonance imaging), 34
MSG (monosodium glutamate), 70, 71, 92
MSM (methylsulfonylmethane), 101
musculoskeletal system, 19–22, 24, 31
MyPyramid, 75

Naproxen (Aleve), 14, 193, 196
National Center for Complementary and Alternative Medicine, 47, 224
National Center for Health Statistics, 210
National Institute of Arthritis and Musculoskeletal and Skin Diseases (NIAMS), 24, 224
National Institutes of Health (NIH), 27, 46–47, 65, 98, 181, 201
neck arthritis, 179, 181, 185, 224
Neck Stretch, 187
*New England Journal of Medicine,* 80
New York Presbyterian Hospital/Weill-Cornell Medical Center, 182